The Complete
Anti-Inflammatory
Diet for Beginners

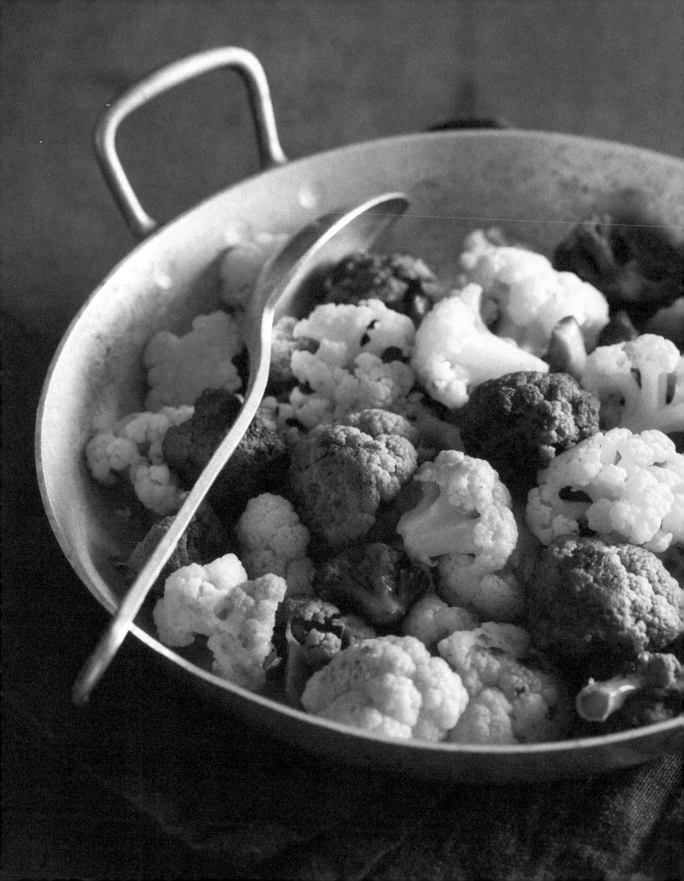

THE COMPLETE
ANTI-INFLAMMATORY
DIET FOR BEGINNERS

A No-Stress Meal Plan
with Easy Recipes to
Heal the Immune System

**Dorothy Calimeris
and Lulu Cook, RDN**

ROCKRIDGE
PRESS

This book is dedicated to readers who are stepping into the market
and into the kitchen to reclaim their good health and well-being —Lulu

This book is for those who want to get the best
from their meals to live a vibrant life. —Dorothy

For general information on our other products and services or to obtain technical support, please contact our Customer Care Department within the US at (866) 744-2665, or outside the US at (510) 253-0500.

Rockridge Press publishes its books in a variety of electronic and print formats. Some content that appears in print may not be available in electronic books, and vice versa.

TRADEMARKS: Rockridge Press and the Rockridge Press logo are trademarks or registered trademarks of Callisto Media Inc. and/or its affiliates, in the United States and other countries, and may not be used without written permission. All other trademarks are the property of their respective owners. Rockridge Press is not associated with any product or vendor mentioned in this book.

Photography © Shannon Douglas, cover; Stockfood/Maike Jessen/Jalag, cover (top right); Stockfood/Olga Miltsova, p. 2; Stockfood/Isolda Delgado Mora, pp. 5, 136 & back cover; Stocksy/Cameron Whitman, pp. 5, 98 & back cover; Stockfood/B.&.E.Dudzinski, pp. 5 & 144; Stockfood/ Victoria Firmston, pp. 6 & 12; Stocksy/Pixel Stories, p. 16; Stocksy/ Susan Brooks-Dammann, p. 17; Stockfood/Jalag/ Janne Peters, p. 26; Stockfood/ Gräfe & Unzer Verlag/ Kramp + Gölling, p. 32; Stockfood/Adrian Britton, p. 38 & back cover; Stockfood/Ursula Schersch, p. 62; Stockfood/ Aniko Szabo, p. 88; Stockfood/Valerie Janssen, p. 108; Stockfood/Hein van Tonder, pp. 120 & 128.

ISBN: Print 978-1-62315-904-7 | eBook 978-1-62315-905-4

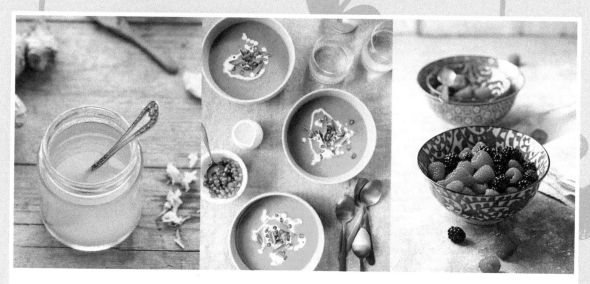

Your Step-by-Step Guide to Anti-Inflammatory Eating

Chronic inflammation does not have to drag you down, sap your energy, or contribute to poor health any longer. You can reverse chronic inflammation through simple dietary changes, and *The Complete Anti-Inflammatory Diet for Beginners* breaks down the process into time-saving, actionable steps.

1. Learn about the diet. Turn to page 16 to learn guidelines for following an anti-inflammatory diet. Discover which foods can soothe inflammation—and worsen it—with the food lists on pages 24 to 25.

2. Plan and prepare your meals. Follow the 2-week meal plan to incorporate healthy cooking into your lifestyle in the most efficient way. With our shopping lists and time-saving suggestions, you can start eating right—right now!

3. Eat, store, and reheat. This plan helps you cook recipes in bulk so you'll have leftovers for lunch or extras to freeze for busy days. The meal plans include tips for repurposing leftovers so you can eat a variety of meals without a lot of extra cooking.

Once you've practiced this healthy cooking method for two weeks, you can repeat the meal plan for a full month of healthy anti-inflammatory eating, or choose from dozens of additional recipes in part 3 for added variety.

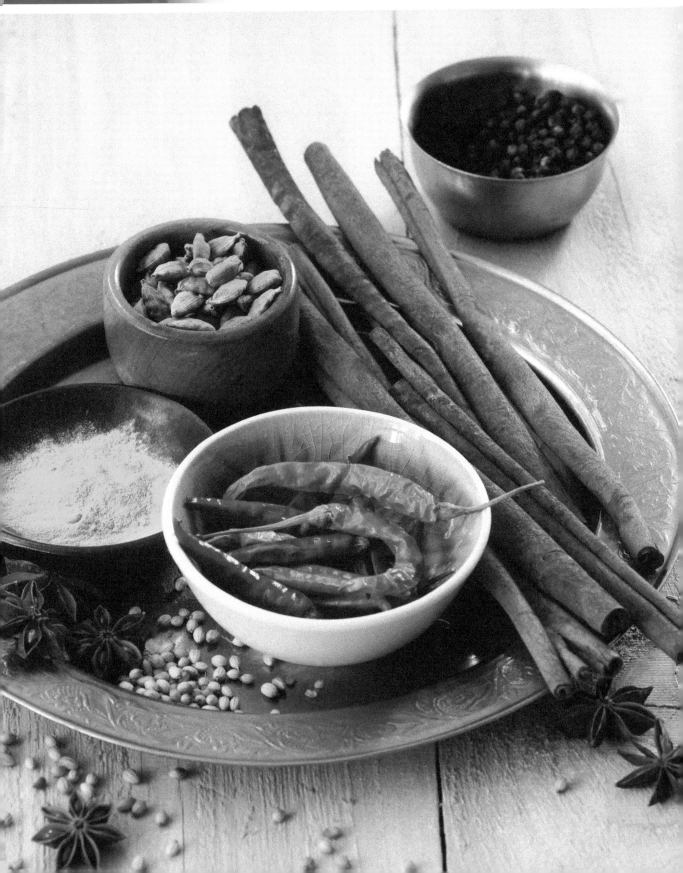

CONTENTS

INTRODUCTION

Lulu's Story

I discovered the power of preparing and eating delicious, nourishing anti-inflammatory meals, when I was an exhausted new mother with a family to feed each night and no idea how to do it. Committed to offering healthy foods to my family, I slowly began to learn about good nutrition. What I noticed first was the positive impact on my energy levels and mood when I ate the way we describe in this book. I just felt better every day, and was able to relax knowing that I was setting my daughter up for a lifetime of good health.

Your sense of vitality, like mine, will increase when you eat foods that promote wellness. I know how challenging it can be to try to make healthy changes, especially when you are already feeling tired, run down, and overworked.

I became a registered dietitian nutritionist to help others access the healing power of whole foods, and to teach people easy ways to incorporate balanced meals into their diets. Since then, I have helped many busy, unhealthy clients who often get stuck in today's hurried ways of eating that leads to chronic inflammation and other diseases. It may seem overwhelming to change your eating lifestyle, but I've heard again and again from people who have reclaimed their own health that the effort is worth it.

It is possible—and really quite simple—to transition to a diet that supports your health goals, by using planning tools and recipes like those we present here. We've broken it down into easy-to-follow steps that provide a broad variety of enjoyable meals. These meals are quick to prepare and just as delicious reheated the next day for something convenient yet nourishing on the go. With these satisfying, tempting foods, you will quickly notice your sense of liveliness and energy increasing, as you begin to live your life with less inflammation and greater gusto!

Dorothy's Story

You may be surprised to hear this, but even those of us who cook for a living are plagued by what to eat, and when to find time to cook! When we're busy and tired, it's all too easy to take the path of least resistance and make poor or impulsive food choices. I have found that planning is the only way to stop this cycle. Every weekend, before I go to the store, I plan my menus for the upcoming week, then I create my shopping list and go to the grocery store. I like to shop on Saturday and cook on Sunday for meals to enjoy all week.

In addition to exploring new recipes that I know will reheat well, I also find it helpful to make batches of simple things like grilled meats, grains, and steamed vegetables for the option of quick salads, stir-fries, or grain bowls so I can have variety and not feel like I'm eating the same thing for lunch and dinner. Although this requires a little advance planning, it saves loads of time later in the week when I don't have time to prep a meal.

As your guide, I have done all the planning and organizing for you, so you can reap the benefits of healthy anti-inflammatory eating with minimal effort. All the recipes are uncomplicated dishes that contain no more than five main ingredients, plus basic pantry staples like cooking oil and dried herbs and spices. These recipes can easily be doubled or tripled to make larger batches to freeze or reheat. As a culinary instructor, I understand that the novice cook may feel overwhelmed or even skeptical, so I've used my experiences to develop a book that guides you, step by step, to plan your meals, cook, and eat in a way that is realistic, manageable, and even fun. This book will help you achieve your goals to eat healthy and feel the best you've felt in ages.

PART ONE

Preparing for the Anti-Inflammatory Diet

The anti-inflammatory diet can be easy, delicious, and affordable—and best of all, it's a great investment in your long-term health and vitality. In this section, we'll lay the foundation to help you better understand how chronic inflammation operates, and explore the tools that will move you toward vibrant well-being. Read on to learn how you can support your body in the healing process through meals that are simple to prepare and satisfying to eat.

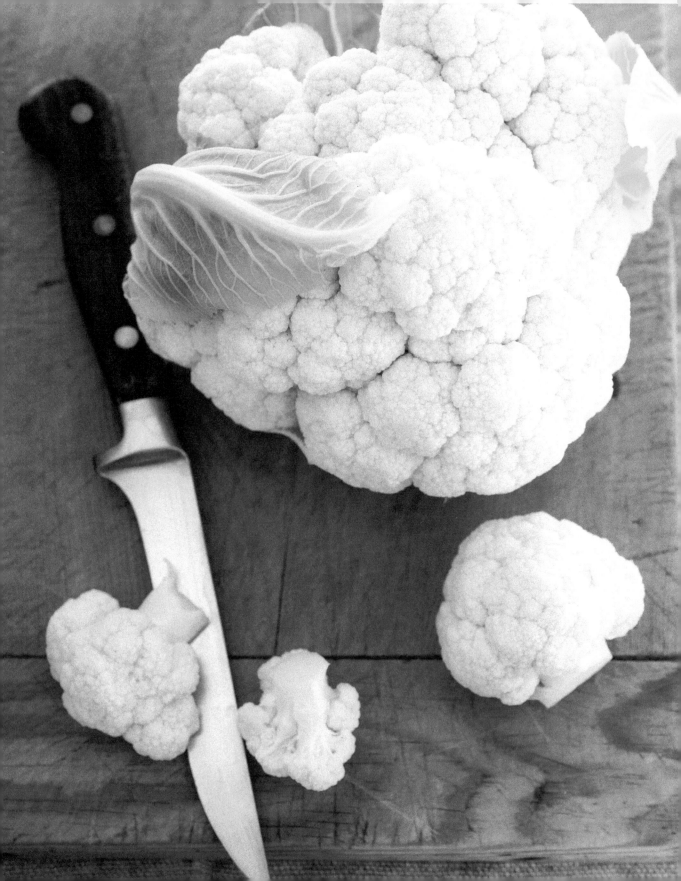

CHAPTER ONE

Anti-Inflammatory Diet Basics

Inflammation can hijack our feelings of wellness and slow us down, but when it becomes chronic, this may signal that something is out of alignment in our diet or lifestyle. Normal inflammation occurs in the body on a regular basis as part of our natural process of maintaining a healthy internal balance. It's only when the necessary process of inflammation gets out of hand that well-being can become impaired. In this chapter, we'll explain how this happens. We'll also present the principles of an easy anti-inflammatory diet, based on whole foods and grounded in science, to support you in restoring your natural balance. Our simple lists of foods to include (and those to avoid) will help you choose meals far beyond the recipes. We'll also touch on how people's bodies respond differently to particular ingredients, so you can personalize these recipes to best meet your own nutritional needs.

How Inflammation Helps—and Harms

When the immune system is working properly, inflammation plays an important role in our body's healthy response to injury or infection. Upon injury or infection, such as a scrape on the knee or exposure to the cold everyone else has at the office, our immune system rallies to restore health. This leads to a period of acute inflammation, which promotes healing as the body's defensive process repairs and restores integrity. Once the problem has been successfully managed, the immune response deactivates, and the inflammation around the area of injury or infection subsides.

When you notice that a paper cut on your finger is red, swollen, warm, and painful, this is all part of inflammation, which is taking place as a result of a smoothly running immune system. Immune cells have been activated to the site of the problem, so blood flow in the area increases, leading to the experience of swelling and heat, which will subside as the wound heals. Soon you'll have nothing to remember the paper cut by but a thin line of scar tissue. This kind of acute, localized inflammation may not require any additional treatment; however, maintaining a consistent anti-inflammatory diet like the one described in this book will ensure that your body has all the nutrients needed to support even this minor healing process.

Conversely, a little cut that seems to hang on too long, remaining puffy and painful and not making much progress in healing, might indicate a bigger issue. In this case, the normal process of acute inflammation may have continued unchecked, signaling a chronic inflammation that is more problematic. This can occur as a result of an unhealed infection like hepatitis B or C, prolonged exposure to environmental toxins like cigarette smoke, or existing health conditions like obesity or auto-immune disease. Lifestyle factors such as diet and stress can also amplify the inflammatory response. At first, there may not be any obvious symptoms of this kind of ongoing low-grade inflammation, yet in the long term, chronic inflammation can increase risk for or exacerbate a variety of diseases.

Recent research has linked chronic inflammation to a wide range of diseases and health conditions, including:

- Obesity
- Type 2 diabetes
- Metabolic syndrome
- Non-alcoholic fatty liver disease
- Some cancers—especially colorectal, gastric, esophageal, pancreatic, breast, endometrial, and ovarian
- Heart/cardiovascular disease
- Hypertension
- Rheumatoid arthritis
- Inflammatory bowel disease
- Crohn's disease
- Ulcerative colitis
- Pancreatitis

Chronic inflammation can cause, exacerbate, or result from these types of health conditions. Repeated or unchecked inflammatory responses play a role in the many complex biological pathways by which disease may result or be worsened. In these disease pathways, protein messengers called cytokines are released as part of the immune response. Some cytokines participate in your body's defensive response to a health threat and accelerate the inflammatory response, while others are anti-inflammatory and help restore balance as you heal. If the balance of proinflammatory to anti-inflammatory cytokines is disrupted, normal cell function can be impaired, and health and well-being may suffer. It can be hard to tell which came first, the inflammation or the disease to which it is linked.

With obesity, for example, a series of causes and effects interact with each other in a downward spiral of declining health. Chronic, low-grade inflammation results directly from consumption of excess calories and obesity. As fat tissue increases, it releases chemicals, hormones, and immune cells that can disrupt normal body function. Proinflammatory cytokines are also released, leading to higher levels of inflammation throughout the body. As the internal system becomes more imbalanced, the risk of developing chronic disorders such as cardiovascular disease, hypertension, type 2 diabetes, and various cancers increases. Many of these conditions increase inflammation themselves. It can become quite complicated when so many of the body's systems are poorly regulated and caught in a feedback loop of actively causing inflammation and damage to other systems.

But there's good news! Consuming anti-inflammatory foods can help straighten out the whole situation, whatever it may be rooted in. An anti-inflammatory diet can support healing if inflammation already exists, and it will provide a foundation for resilience in the future.

Shift your focus to this kind of nourishing, balanced, and tasty diet and you'll see a difference in no time, as this diet will restore the energy and sense of well-being you deserve.

Principles of the Anti-Inflammatory Diet

Experts agree that a diet consisting of a wide range of plant-based foods, accompanied by moderate amounts of whole grains, lean proteins, and healthful fats, is the type of eating pattern that will reduce inflammation and ensure a robust immune system. We are constantly learning more about the negative effects of heavily processed, packaged foods, which are often high in inflammation-promoting sodium, added sugars, refined grains, and detrimental fats. Conversely, this book emphasizes fresh, whole foods that are prepared using healthy cooking techniques. Vibrant herbs and spices are not just good for punching up flavor—you'll learn how each brings its own health-supportive qualities to your meals. Prebiotic and probiotic foods support your microbiome—that's the name for the beneficial gut bacteria in your digestive system. These bacteria are linked to a thriving immune system. And you can wash it all down with powerful inflammation-fighting beverages such as unsweetened tea and coffee, water infused with herbs or fruit (see Own Your Water, page 19), and the occasional glass of red wine, if you choose to partake.

We present recipes inspired by the many traditional cuisines around the world that

ANTI-INFLAMMATORY DIET GUIDELINES

Eat more plants. Explore and enjoy the wide range of fruits and vegetables that provide fiber, antioxidants, and other nutrients to support optimal health. These low-calorie foods combat cellular damage, promote digestion, and help maintain a healthy weight range, which keeps inflammation in check as well.

Discover whole and ancient grains. Ancient grains are those that predate modern varieties created through selective breeding and hybridization—think oats, barley, chia, sorghum, quinoa, bulgur, and the like. These and whole grains retain fiber, antioxidants, and other nutrients that promote

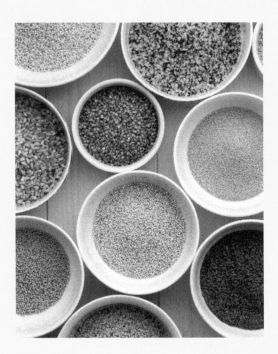

a healthy immune response. If whole grains are new to you, try mixing them 50/50 with your usual choice to begin dining the anti-inflammatory way, such as white rice with brown rice, quinoa with couscous, or whole-wheat bread crumbs with white.

Choose healthy fats. Plant-based options like olive oil contain unsaturated fats that support immunity. These are preferable to proinflammatory trans fats and saturated fats from animal products, like butter and bacon. Look for omega-3 fats, such as fish and walnuts, to directly reduce inflammation.

Enjoy nuts and seeds. These little bites provide healthy fats and protein, as well as valuable micronutrients and fiber. Plus, their flavor and crunch enhance any meal or snack.

Add flavor with herbs and spices. Turmeric, ginger, and garlic are anti-inflammatory powerhouses. Have fun exploring these and countless other options for their deep flavors and unique benefits.

Support your microbiome. High-fiber foods like beans and whole grains provide nourishment for your beneficial gut bacteria to thrive. Fermented foods such as yogurt, kimchi, and pickles keep the "communities" of bacteria in your digestive system balanced to help fight inflammation and disease.

Consume power beverages. Coffee and unsweetened black or green tea offer antioxidant compounds that promote resilience against cell damage. Enjoy red wine on occasion, if you like, to maximize anti-inflammatory benefits. Plain water is always a great choice for keeping your body hydrated and energized—vary the flavor and benefits by tossing in some cut fruit or herbs (see Own Your Water, page 19).

Eat fewer processed foods. Highly processed foods are often high in added sugars, refined grains, sodium, and detrimental fats. These types of foods are proinflammatory and also increase one's risk for weight gain and other diseases. If you haven't yet, become a label reader to increase your awareness of what's in these foods—it may surprise and inspire you to run toward the whole foods sections of the store.

Consume less meat. When you want meat, choose and prepare it carefully. Many meats have undesirable amounts of unhealthy fats, and some are pumped full of sodium during processing. Use cooking methods that do not blacken the meat, such as grilling, as the blackened parts that occur have compounds that can contribute to inflammation.

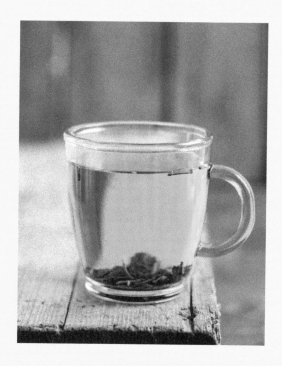

Relax! Stress is a significant contributor to inflammation and disease—in fact, chronic elevation of the stress hormone cortisol leads to ongoing negative impacts on health. Get more sleep, boost your physical activity, and try new activities such as mindfulness meditation—these all help manage stress and keep inflammation down.

promote a vigorous immune response. Traditional Japanese diets, for instance, are low in fat and full of nutrient-rich vegetables and seafood, but contain very little sugar or refined flour. A modified paleo approach is also explored here, including generous portions of vegetables and hearty protein dishes prepared from the healthiest meats. The Mediterranean eating pattern is well studied for its anti-inflammatory, health-promoting qualities, and many people find its familiar flavors satisfying and appealing. It is based on abundant fruits and vegetables, along with whole grains, legumes, and nuts. Fish, red wine, and olive oil are incorporated regularly in Mediterranean cooking, while red meat, added sugars, and high-fat dairy are limited. We are inspired by this delicious style of eating, so you'll see a lot of recipes here that reflect the Mediterranean approach. But we also recognize that the only anti-inflammatory diet that will work for you is the one you find satisfying and delicious. So after you master the basics, use these principles to figure out which styles you enjoy best and fine-tune your own anti-inflammatory lifestyle path!

Smart Dietary Choices

A whole foods approach to eating is the best route to decreasing inflammation, and that's the strategy we present here. As the benefits of anti-inflammatory diets become clearer, a growing number of studies reveal which foods are best to include or avoid as you move toward vibrant wellness. Let's check them out.

Foods That Fight Inflammation

FRUITS AND VEGETABLES. Consider yourself free to enjoy a wide range of fruits and vegetables on the anti-inflammatory diet—they're all good! Plant foods deliver a high-nutrient, low-calorie foundation and add bright, tempting color to any plate. These foods are a source of satisfying, anti-inflammatory fiber, plus vitamins, minerals, and micronutrients. Fruits and vegetables also contain powerful antioxidant compounds that help prevent cellular damage.

Berries, watermelon, apples, and pineapple in particular are proven anti-inflammatory superstars, thanks to their high levels of phytonutrients. Thousands of these chemicals can be found in different combinations in plant foods, and while they protect the plant against environmental damage, they also protect you on a cellular level, especially when you eat a wide range of produce. Citrus fruits provide high-antioxidant vitamin C, a knockout inflammation fighter. Vegetables such as onions, broccoli, and leafy greens support resistance to inflammation. Garlic and onion don't just add pungent flavor—they've also been studied extensively for their immune system benefits.

NIGHTSHADES. Beware the boundless Internet (mis)information available—some is inaccurate and not well grounded in science. Rumors that you can't enjoy nightshades such as tomatoes, potatoes, bell peppers, and eggplant on an anti-inflammatory diet are unfounded for most people. While some with autoimmune conditions like rheumatoid arthritis choose to avoid these nutritious vegetables, the Arthritis Foundation notes that no scientific data supports this, and in fact, the group cites research that shows that consumption of yellow and purple potatoes may actually lower inflammation. However, you are the expert of your own body. If you find that this restriction is supportive of your own health and well-being, then just try to include a wide range of other vegetables to ensure you are providing all the nutrition your body needs to heal. For most people, nightshade vegetables are part of a nutritious, anti-inflammatory diet. For instance, compounds such as the lycopene provided by cooked tomatoes make these vegetables standouts for fighting inflammation.

WHOLE AND ANCIENT GRAINS. Whole and ancient grains don't merely replace refined grains. They provide exciting flavors and textures, along with fiber, micronutrients, antioxidants, and protein. Naturally gluten-free grains, such as quinoa and amaranth, keep meals interesting and can be enjoyed by everyone.

GOOD FATS. We have learned that it's more important to enjoy the right kinds of fats in moderation than to try to eliminate fat altogether. Olive oil is a rich source of polyphenols, which are compounds shown to reduce indicators of inflammation, and it should be your primary cooking oil. Specialty oils like walnut oil or pumpkin seed oil add rich flavor and beneficial unsaturated fats. And we're happy to promote the benefits of dark chocolate, a delicious source of protective polyphenols— and a fine end to a meal!

OMEGA-3 FATTY ACIDS ARE ALL-STAR ANTI-INFLAMMATORY FATS. Include foods with this type of unsaturated fat frequently to optimize your whole diet approach. Fatty fish like salmon and sardines are excellent sources, as are some plant foods such as walnuts and flaxseed. Flaxseed may sound foreign, but it's been around for thousands of years, just now gaining popularity for its abundant fiber, protein, and powerful antioxidants called lignans.

OWN YOUR WATER

Water can be the most refreshing treat when you're parched. A decanter of water with sliced cucumber in a hotel lobby is a welcome sight to weary travelers. Yet it's amazing to see how many people have a hard time taking in enough water each day. If you're one of them, consider adding some fruits or herbs to your water to boost the flavor and the benefits. Buy a pretty glass pitcher; it will make the water look especially inviting. Ginger, thyme, basil, and rosemary make good herbal anti-inflammatory add-ins; beneficial fruits include orange, grapefruit, lemon, lime, apples, watermelon, and pineapple. Try water infused with blueberries and lemon, cucumber and mint, or beets and rosemary—or come up with your own favorite flavor combinations!

Consumption of flaxseed protects against inflammation and some cancers, but go for the ground version, so your body can absorb all that goodness. Seeds like hemp and chia are similarly helpful, as are pine nuts, which are actually nutrient-dense seeds.

HERBS AND SPICES. With countless options, each herb and spice has a unique profile of antioxidants and bright flavors to complement all kinds of cuisine. Turmeric deserves special mention for its proven anti-inflammatory and neuroprotective properties. Ginger, saffron, and cinnamon are other potent flavor enhancers worth trying. Herbs such as basil, rosemary, and thyme all have inflammation-fighting compounds, and their aroma and taste elevate the meal experience.

PROBIOTICS AND PREBIOTICS. What are these, anyway? Probiotics and prebiotics support immune and digestive health. Fermented foods such as yogurt, sauerkraut, pickles, tempeh, and kimchi are known as probiotic foods because they provide a direct infusion of healthy bacteria to your system in addition to their characteristic tang. Prebiotics are foods that feed those good gut bacteria—sources include high-fiber vegetables, whole grains, and beans. Cooked beans like black beans, chickpeas, and lentils also double as lean, plant-based proteins.

HEALTHY DRINKS. Washing foods down with kombucha keeps the probiotic theme going, although not everyone appreciates the sour taste of this fermented beverage! Thankfully, unsweetened teas are good beverage options— green tea is a particularly robust source of antioxidants. Drip coffee provides fiber and is one of the biggest contributors of anti-oxidants to the American diet—just try to keep it sugar-free. A glass of red wine from time to time provides protective resveratrol. Water is always a great choice for hydration (see Own Your Water, page 19) and promotes the body's ability to detoxify at the cellular level.

Foods That Worsen Inflammation

PROCESSED FOODS. There is no shortage of delicious, nourishing food to enjoy on your anti-inflammatory diet. To maximize the benefits, you'll want to leave behind those highly processed, packaged foods, as they are typically full of proinflammatory sodium, saturated fats, added sugars, and refined grains such as white flour or white rice.

AVOID ADDED SUGARS AND REFINED GRAINS FROM ANY SOURCE. These proinflammatory foods dramatically increase blood sugar, have more calories than they do nutrition, and are linked to many negative health effects.

PROCESSED AND RED MEAT. Some meats, such as ham and many deli meats, are highly processed and contain undesirable saturated fat and sodium. Red meat is another food to choose less frequently. Even lean cuts are likely to have high levels of proinflammatory saturated fats. You might be surprised to know that you should save backyard cookouts for special occasions. This is because fatty proteins like beef prepared with high-heat dry cooking methods increase production of proinflammatory substances called advanced glycation end products, or AGEs. Consider using lower-heat, moist cooking methods, such as stewing, sautéing, or poaching, to minimize this effect. Select lean, grass-fed beef options that offer protective omega-3s, in contrast with regular beef, which is high in proinflammatory omega-6 fats.

Foods to Consider with Care

Many foods fall in the middle of the health spectrum—these foods are neither the foundation of an anti-inflammatory diet nor the worst choices. These should be considered with care, depending on your own goals and current health condition. These foods are used sparingly in our recipes, and when we do include them, we offer substitutions.

CERTAIN OILS. A few plant-based oils should be approached thoughtfully. Corn, safflower, sunflower, and soy oils are high in proinflammatory omega-6s. Despite the trendiness of coconut oil on websites that promise "magic results" from consuming it in high amounts, it is a highly saturated fat, and there is no reason to believe it is healthy to consume in excess. Occasional dishes can be prepared with coconut oil, but keep olive oil as your go-to kitchen staple.

SKIN-ON DARK-MEAT POULTRY AND PORK. Skinless white-meat poultry can serve as a good source of protein. However, higher-fat dark meat and poultry with skin-on are less healthful. Many pork products contain too much fat and sodium to belong in an anti-inflammatory diet, but very lean pork, such as pork tenderloin, can be enjoyed occasionally.

NATURAL SUGARS. We all deserve a treat, and nobody wants to feel deprived. When your sweet tooth does strike, the best sweets to choose, in moderation, are natural sugars such as honey, maple syrup, and molasses rather than refined sugar products. These offer some trace micronutrients, along with the sweet taste we crave.

Unique Bodies, Unique Reactions to Food

We also treat the "Big 8" food allergens (fish, shellfish, peanuts, tree nuts, wheat, soy, eggs, and dairy) as "Consider with Care" foods, to highlight them for those individuals who need to make substitutions. Food allergies are immune system responses in which the body mistakenly responds to proteins, in otherwise wholesome foods, as a threat. Food allergies can be life threatening, and those with food allergies know they must be vigilant to ensure they are not accidentally consuming foods that will stimulate a negative immune response.

Some people have sensitivities and intolerances to particular foods that are not technically allergies, as they do not involve the immune system. The research into this area is growing but still inconclusive; for many individuals, the best barometer for food tolerance comes from simply paying attention to how you feel after consuming that food. You know your own body best, so please modify the diet we present here to your needs. If you are uncertain about how well a particular food fits into your own dietary pattern, keep note of how you react when you eat that food, and consider consulting with a registered dietitian.

For those who can consume fish and shellfish, these are potent inflammation fighters. Deep-water fish offer unparalleled amounts of omega-3 fats in a form that is very easy for the body to use in fighting inflammation, so salmon and herring can be regular staples of your diet if you are not allergic.

Peanuts and tree nuts (walnuts, cashews, etc.) are anti-inflammatory powerhouses. If you're able to eat them, small portions of almonds or pecans provide the antioxidant vitamin E, healthy fats, and a bit of protein in addition to their rich, satisfying crunch.

Most people can consume nutritious ancient grains with no problems. If you have celiac disease or are intolerant or allergic to gluten, you'll want to avoid wheat berries and barley. Ancient grains may be avoided on strict elimination diets, which are not necessary for most people wanting to reduce inflammation. We also list the more processed whole-grain products under "Consider with Care." Whole-wheat bread is a step in the right direction from white bread, but it is still highly processed. Intact whole grains such as quinoa reign supreme for their anti-inflammatory power.

Soy is a major allergen but also a powerful inflammation fighter. Despite widespread myths, research shows that soy reduces inflammation and cancer risks for most people—great news if you enjoy popping steamed edamame in your mouth at your favorite sushi restaurant! Soy is a high-protein source of fiber, so unless you have an allergy, freely include edamame and tofu in your diet.

Eggs offer micronutrients such as choline and lutein, but they're another common allergen. While they do not appear to have specifically anti-inflammatory properties, they can serve as a good protein source in a healthy, balanced diet. If you can, consider including eggs as part of your overall dietary strategy.

Dairy is another major food allergen. Low- or non-fat dairy products, and those cultured to provide probiotics, like yogurt and kefir, should be considered with care. There is controversy over the benefits of including full-fat dairy in one's diet, but in relation to inflammation, the picture is clearer. Sources of saturated fat, like butter and cream, are best limited on an anti-inflammatory diet, so we don't use them here.

Anti-Inflammatory Food Lists

Foods in the "Enjoy" section (page 24) can be eaten freely by most people. Challenge yourself to try them all! "Consider with Care" foods are nutritious for many people to consume as part of an otherwise balanced meal pattern. If you have a food allergy or other health consideration, choose one of the other options provided. The "Avoid" foods promote inflammation and can derail your efforts. Look for ways to swap those out for foods on the "Enjoy" list!

Benefits You'll See

Change can be hard—even positive change! As you begin this diet, you may find yourself challenged as you begin thinking about your meal choices in unfamiliar ways. That's a great reason to use the shopping lists and meal plans as we've presented them. This will take the guesswork and decision making out of the early stages of your transition to an anti-inflammatory lifestyle. Then you'll build confidence to begin testing out variations that work for you.

At first, you will notice that you are satisfied after each meal or snack, and that the energy you feel is more lasting throughout your day. You may find yourself getting hungry less often; this is because you're consuming more nutrient-dense foods. You may even see your skin clearing up as you remove highly processed foods and added sugars and replace them with more nourishing options that support health at the cellular level. Many people who shift to this eating style report gradual weight loss over time, which is also beneficial for reducing inflammation.

Less visible but equally important are the longer-term improvements you may notice in your health. If you happen to get a blood test from your doctor, you'll probably see the markers of inflammation, such as C-reactive protein (CRP) and interleukin 6 (IL-6), going down, and a more healthy lipid profile—higher HDL ("good") cholesterol and lower LDL ("bad") cholesterol—emerging over time. Your energy will likely be increasingly vibrant yet grounded and calm, and your body will be better able to fight off infection, whether that means just a little cold or a more significant threat. Your energy will increase, you will be better equipped to manage stress, and you'll just feel better—all qualities that can't be quantified in a lab test. Rather, you'll notice it when you bound out of bed in the morning, feeling great and ready to tackle the day—after a nourishing and satisfying anti-inflammatory breakfast, that is!

FOODS TO ENJOY

VEGETABLES (FRESH, FROZEN, OR CANNED WITHOUT ADDED SODIUM)

Alliums
Chives
Garlic*
Leeks
Onions*
Scallions
Shallots

Cruciferous Vegetables*
Arugula
Bok choy
Broccoli
Brussels sprouts
Cabbage
Cauliflower
Collard greens
Kale
Kohlrabi
Mizuna
Mustard greens
Radish greens
Romanesco broccoli/
Roman cauliflower
Turnip greens

Dark Green Leafy Vegetables
Lettuces, especially romaine*
Spinach*
Swiss chard*

Root Vegetables
Beets
Carrots
Celery root/celeriac
Radishes
Rutabagas
Sweet potatoes
Turnips
Winter squash

Other Vegetables
Asparagus
Bell peppers
Corn
Fermented, probiotic vegetables*
Green beans
Mushrooms

FRUIT (FRESH, FROZEN, OR CANNED WITHOUT ADDED SUGAR)

Apples
Apricots
Avocados
Bananas
Berries*
Citrus*
Cranberries

Figs
Grapes
Kiwi
Mangos
Melons
Pineapple*
Stone fruit

FATS AND OILS

Nut oils
Olive oil*

Seed oils

WHOLE AND ANCIENT GRAINS

Amaranth*
Brown rice
Buckwheat*
Millet*

Oatmeal*
Popcorn
Quinoa*
Teff*

SEEDS

Chia
Flaxseed*
Hemp
Mustard

Poppy
Pumpkin
Sesame
Sunflower

HERBS AND SPICES

Basil
Bay leaf
Cilantro
Cinnamon*
Clove
Dill
Ginger*
Mint
Nutmeg
Oregano*

Paprika
Parsley
Pepper
Rosemary*
Saffron*
Sage
Tarragon
Thyme
Turmeric*

PROTEINS

Beans*
Tempeh*

Tofu

OTHER

Unsweetened coffee

Unsweetened black or green tea*

Note: Asterisks indicate foods that are particularly beneficial anti-inflammatory superstars.

CONSIDER WITH CARE

FATS AND OILS

Coconut	Sesame
Corn	Soy
Safflower	Sunflower

WHOLE AND ANCIENT GRAINS

Barley	Spelt
Emmer	Wheat berries
Farro	Whole-grain breads, bulgur, couscous, pastas
Rye	

NUTS AND SEEDS

Peanuts	Tree nuts* (e.g., almonds, cashews, macadamias, pistachios, walnuts*)

DAIRY

Fermented, probiotic dairy* (e.g., kefir, yogurt)	Low-fat and non-fat dairy products (e.g., cheese, milk)

PROTEINS

Eggs	Poultry (skinless white meat)
Fish* (e.g., cod, flounder, halibut, mackerel, salmon,* sardines,* tuna)	Shellfish (e.g., mussels, oysters, scallops)
Pork (very lean cuts, such as pork tenderloin)	Soy (e.g., edamame/soybeans, tofu, tempeh)

OTHER

Dark chocolate	Red wine

AVOID

FATS AND OILS

Butter	Margarine
Lard	

GRAINS

All refined grains (e.g., white bread and rolls, white pasta, white rice)	Packaged, processed grain-based snacks and desserts (e.g., biscuits, cakes, cereals, cookies, crackers, muffins)
	Pastries

OTHER

Bacon	High-sodium foods
Beef (especially high-fat cuts, beef charred on the grill, and corn-fed beef—typically any that is not grass-fed)	Packaged and processed foods
	Packaged, processed meat alternatives (e.g., "garden burgers," faux chicken)
Full-fat dairy (e.g., butter, cheese, cream, half-and-half, ice cream)	Refined added sugars (brown sugar, confectioners' sugar, high-fructose corn syrup, white sugar)
High-fat foods (especially those with high saturated fats or trans fats)	

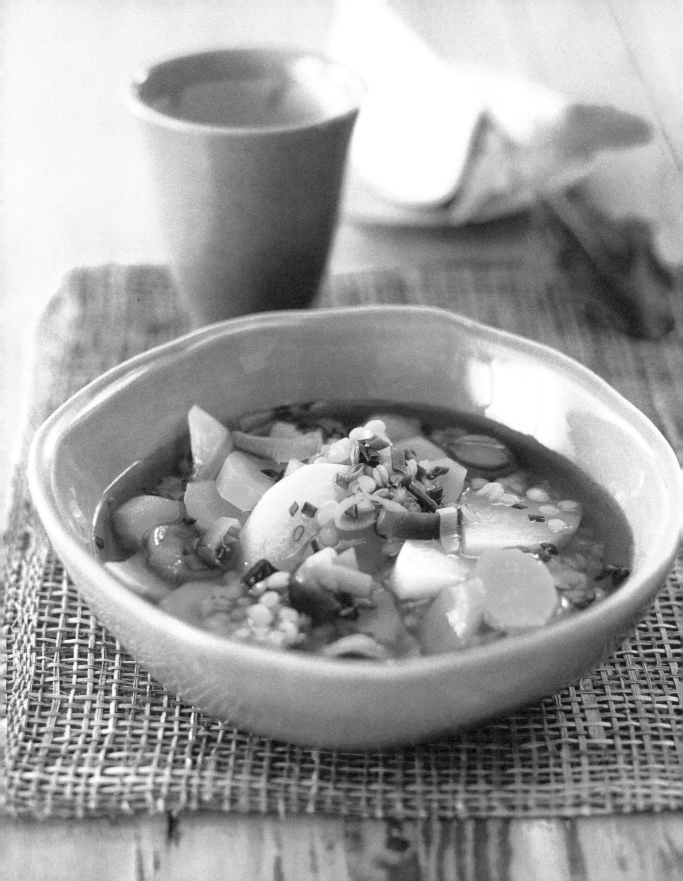

CHAPTER TWO

Preparing for a Healthy Change

Now that you know how inflammatory processes can help *and* hinder, it's time to move toward your mission to reduce chronic inflammation and reclaim your energy and vitality. Here you'll learn how to harness the right mindset and some lifestyle measures you can take outside of the kitchen to optimize your plan. You don't have to tackle them all at once. Select just one or two to start—this will set the foundation for success and enhance your sense of well-being right away! You'll find action steps and practical information in this chapter as well, such as the tools and equipment you'll need to get your kitchen and pantry ready. The productivity hacks you'll find here are the final secret weapons for easy and convenient preparation of appealing, satisfying anti-inflammatory meals to enjoy both at home and on the go.

A Positive Mindset

An anti-inflammatory diet can be fun, delicious, and empowering . . . or it can seem overwhelming and restrictive. To achieve success and have some fun doing it, first stop and consider the mindset you bring to this transition. Then cultivate approaches that keep your motivation high.

One way to support yourself is by practicing mindfulness. Mindfulness is a way of paying attention to what you are experiencing in each moment. Thoughts like "I don't have time to take care of myself with nourishing foods," or "I never make good choices," can derail you in reaching your goals, but when you become aware of these kinds of completely normal but self-defeating thoughts, you have more power over them. Self-compassion can begin to free you from old ways of thinking. Instead of following through on those negative thoughts automatically, decide to veto your thoughts and choose a different course of action.

How does this work in regard to eating? In this case, mindfulness helps you gain insight into how you talk to yourself and the impulses driving your eating choices. This exercise will support you in breaking old habits and transitioning to foods that keep you fueled in a sustained and lasting way. And it will eventually become natural. Imagine how great you will feel in light of all this positive change—you broke old habits, achieved success, and improved your health! As time goes on, your mindfulness practice will help you be more aware of how energized and steady you feel when you nourish yourself this way.

By taking time to sit and thoughtfully enjoy your food, you can use mindful eating as a way to check in with yourself anytime you eat. It becomes a more powerful tool when you practice it regularly.

Retrain Your Brain to Look at the Bright Side

Did you know that our brains are naturally designed to respond more strongly to unpleasant stimuli than to pleasant ones and to notice (and remember) negative experiences more than positive ones? This phenomenon, known as negativity bias, made sense in the early days of civilization because giving more mental weight to things that seem dangerous or frightening helped us survive as a species, by priming us to take action in the face of potential threats. It was less important to pay attention to things that were merely pleasant. In modern life, this means that experiences that are challenging, such as transitioning to a new way of eating, can take up more brain space than experiences that are easy and familiar. Our brains get hijacked by alarm bells in the face of difficult stimuli, and we lose the ability to make careful, discerning choices about how to think, act, and eat.

Being aware of this challenge can help you maintain a positive attitude. Remind yourself that it's natural to feel skeptical or negative about shifting established habits, even when it's to benefit your health. You can reframe this negativity bias by finding ways to appreciate the positive aspects of your new lifestyle. Include gratitude in your mindfulness practice by focusing on the delicious new flavors you are exploring or your success in creating the recipes. Notice and really savor neutral and positive experiences for at least 6 to 12 seconds, the time it takes for an experience to enter our long-term memory, and do this as often as you can every day. By purposefully keeping your attention on the present moment, you're training your brain to amplify the bright side, rather than just dwelling on the negative.

Ready, Set, Go!

You can start some aspects of an anti-inflammatory lifestyle right away, while giving yourself time to prepare. It takes a while to establish new habits, so use this week to get organized.

DAY 1: TAKE NOTES. Begin increasing your awareness of what you eat. The best way to do this is by keeping a food journal—simply note and record what, when, and how much you eat. Research shows that keeping a food journal leads to healthier eating behaviors, even without intentionally making different choices. It does not need to be fancy—you can use a notebook or a tracking app like Lose It. Just snapping a picture of your food with a cell phone is enough to increase awareness.

DAY 2: PRACTICE MINDFUL EATING. Mindful eating is a way of staying present with what you are eating and realizing how it affects you. Spend this day paying attention and tasting every bite fully, then noticing how it impacts your energy and well-being. First, turn off the television and step away from the electronics! Take a moment to close your eyes and notice how hungry you are, as well as any other sensations you may be feeling. Put a bite of food in

your mouth and chew slowly, paying attention to the texture and taste without distraction. Continue eating in this way, noticing each bite and how your body is feeling. It's the most delicious way to practice meditation!

DAY 3: GET SMART. Choose SMART goals as you transition to an anti-inflammatory lifestyle—that is, Specific, Measurable, Achievable, Realistic, and Time-limited. These kinds of actions should be within your power to accomplish. For instance, a SMART goal for anti-inflammatory eating might be, "I will print the shopping list from this book and go to the grocery store on Sunday afternoon to purchase items I need for the week." Use today to reflect on your motivation for reducing chronic inflammation, then write down your SMART goals to help cement your commitment.

DAY 4: MAP OUT A PLAN. With your SMART goals in hand, look at your calendar and map out how you are going to transition to the anti-inflammatory diet. Decide when you will go to the store. You may want to make a game plan for special events and trips, as well as any modifications to adapt the program to your specific dietary needs. Looking ahead in your calendar can help you plan for any challenges that might otherwise trip you up.

DAY 5: TELL ON YOURSELF. Share your goals with someone you trust. Enlist that person to help keep you on track in a way that is useful for you. Some people benefit from the accountability of reporting regularly to a friend about their progress. Others just want to know they have an ally to turn to if any challenges arise. Identify someone who will cheer you on when you nail your goals. Having social support has been shown to help people achieve success in transitioning to healthier behaviors, so take advantage of this tool.

DAY 6: LOOK AT THE BIGGER PICTURE. Don't think of the anti-inflammatory diet as achievement of some ideal of perfection. It's more about consciously redirecting your eating patterns to reduce chronic inflammation over time—a more forgiving mindset. You have every right to ground your commitment in the realistic acknowledgement that "Hey, sometimes I'm going to have that slice of birthday cake with my family." Just plan in advance to help you decide what you will do in those situations. Imagine what it will be like to have an overall nourishing diet, while mindfully enjoying an occasional indulgence—a much more achievable mindset than zeroing in on every single bite with a "make it or break it" attitude! And when slip-ups occur, rather than beat yourself up, acknowledge that it happened, commit to try better next time, and then return your attention to the bigger picture and the sustainable power of your positive meal choices over the long term.

DAY 7: GIVE IT 30 DAYS. You may wonder, when will this new lifestyle feel natural? Research shows it can take 30 to 60 days to establish new habits. You may have days when you feel fantastic. You may also have days when it takes a lot of effort to stick with this new lifestyle. Expect things to seem unfamiliar and challenging at first, with moments when you just want to slide into old debilitating habits—this is natural. These are good times to practice mindful self-compassion, and to reach out to one of your cheerleaders who can encourage you to stay resolute. Remember your long-term goals and celebrate the little successes along the way, and you will build new habits and experience renewed and vibrant health that makes any short-term discomfort more than worthwhile.

The Anti-Inflammatory Kitchen and Pantry

Now that we've discussed the right mindset for your new diet, let's move this party into the kitchen. Since desperation is the mother of invention, please don't feel that you need to go purchase everything on this list of tools. Any item that gets the job done is adequate—for instance, a spent gift card makes a splendid bowl scraper! However, we've listed some of the equipment and pantry items you may find useful to have on hand.

Kitchen Equipment and Tools

- A variety of knives (paring, chef's, serrated)
- Long-handled wooden spoons
- Heat-resistant spatulas
- Tongs
- 10-inch (or so) skillet
- Baking sheet
- Mixing bowls
- Potato masher
- Dutch oven
- Slow cooker
- Blender and/or food processor
- Single-serving food storage containers
- Quart-size food storage containers

Your Basic Anti-Inflammatory Pantry

DRIED HERBS AND SPICES
- Cardamom, ground
- Chipotle powder
- Cinnamon, ground
- Cumin, ground
- Curry powder
- Garlic powder
- Ginger, ground
- Mustard, ground
- Nutmeg, ground
- Onion powder
- Oregano, dried
- Peppercorns, black
- Rosemary, dried
- Sage, dried
- Sea salt
- Turmeric, ground

GLUTEN-FREE FLOURS AND GRAINS
- Almond meal or flour
- Brown rice
- Buckwheat groats
- Coconut flour
- Oats
- Quinoa
- Wild rice

CANNED, JARRED, AND BAGGED FOODS
- Black beans
- Chicken broth, low-sodium
- Chickpeas
- Coconut milk, unsweetened
- Lentils
- Vegetable broth, low-sodium

OILS AND VINEGARS
- Almond oil
- Apple cider vinegar
- Balsamic vinegar
- Coconut oil
- Extra-virgin olive oil
- Sesame oil

NONDAIRY MILK
- Almond milk, unsweetened
- Coconut milk, unsweetened
- Rice milk, unsweetened

SWEETENERS
- Honey, raw
- Maple syrup

MISCELLANEOUS
- Baking powder
- Baking soda
- Dijon mustard (no added sugar)
- Vanilla extract

Cooking with Efficiency

There are a million formulas for efficient planning, and you'll soon discover your favorites. Figure out your best days to shop and cook, and schedule them on your calendar. You might want to shop one day and bulk-cook the next—that way, everything you need will be on hand so you can focus on prepping and cooking.

If you find it overwhelming to map out a week's worth of meals at once, you can plan on

ARSENAL OF TIME-SAVING TOOLS

Here are six pieces of equipment you won't want to live without!

Slow cooker. The slow cooker has been around for a long time and isn't particularly exciting, but it's a workhorse that allows you to come home to a fully cooked dinner. You might want to use your slow cooker on the weekends to help create meals for the week ahead.

Cast-iron skillet. This good old-fashioned piece of equipment can go from stove to oven, giving you one less pot or pan to wash. They're inexpensive and last forever.

Vegetable chopper. If you're not comfortable using a knife, buy an inexpensive vegetable chopper. Simply cut the vegetables so they fit in the chopper, attach the lid, and press the plunger to begin chopping. This manual gadget is perfect for chopping onions, garlic, carrots, and celery for soups and sauces. It's also useful if you have a small kitchen with no space for a large cutting board.

Canning jars. Quality food storage containers can be expensive, and if you send a guest home with leftovers, the containers probably won't come back. Instead, consider using canning jars—they're inexpensive and easy to find, and they take up minimal space in the refrigerator or freezer. They're also easy to fill with leftovers for tomorrow's lunch.

Insulated shopping bag. An insulated bag is ideal for purchasing food and keeping it fresh until you get home, as well as for taking prepared food and snacks on road trips.

Low-profile blender. A small blender—either an immersion blender or a smoothie blender—comes in handy for many kitchen tasks. It takes up very little space in the kitchen and can be used to purée soups and sauces, blend smoothies, purée salad dressing, or, in the case of the smoothie blender, make pestos and other herb sauces.

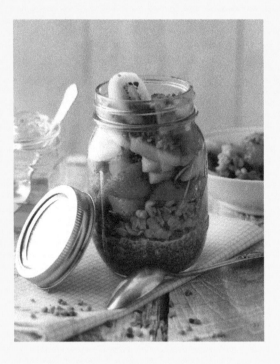

just three days' worth of meals at a time. Then just schedule another shopping trip mid-week, utilizing healthy prepared foods like whole roast chickens, bagged greens, and steamed, unseasoned vegetables sold in the hot food or deli section of the market. You'll come to know which stores stock the best prepared meals, and which you prefer.

When you come home from shopping, clean and prep your vegetables as you put them away. You can ask the bagger at the market to put all your produce in one or two bags. After putting the other groceries away, tackle your produce bag—wash, peel, chop, and transfer to food storage containers. It is so satisfying to peek in the refrigerator and see those colorful prepped veggies all ready to pop into a pan!

If time is more of an issue than budget, take advantage of the already prepped and chopped items available at the store—they are usually more expensive than the whole versions. Many stores carry chopped fresh vegetables, including butternut squash, carrots, onions, celery, beets, zucchini, and cauliflower. More stores are adding prepped organic vegetables to their produce offerings as well. When time is tight, your commitment to healthy eating need not suffer with so many convenient options.

Another good strategy to ensure efficiency is to review the week's recipes before you begin cooking, and do as much of the prep ahead of time as possible. Gather your ingredients and consider how you can be efficient while prepping. For example, if two recipes call for chopped onions, then chop enough for both recipes, or if three recipes call for cooked chicken, cook enough chicken for all three and divide it among the recipes. Start with ingredients that take longer to cook first—like boiled eggs—and chop your vegetables while the eggs are cooking. Try to challenge yourself to cook as if you're putting a puzzle together. How can I organize myself so everything is done on time and made with a minimum number of pots and pans?

When you're putting dinner leftovers away, use this opportunity to pack lunch for the next day. It makes a world of difference when you're rushing to work in the morning. In addition to getting your entrée ready, also pack some fruit and anything else you're taking, so it's all ready to go.

Lastly, if you know you have a crazy week ahead, plan anti-inflammatory dining out or taking in. Review the menus of your favorite restaurants online before you go, and choose the best anti-inflammatory options. A little planning will support your body through its stressful week while helping maintain your health goals.

Tips for Storing and Reheating Food

- Storing and reheating food well is important for safety reasons, and it can keep those leftovers flavorful and appealing to eat.
- Allow food to cool completely before placing it in storage containers.
- Use containers with tight-fitting lids, such as canning jars, or plastic containers.
- Ideally, portion food into single servings for quick reheating.
- Most foods will last for up to five days in the refrigerator or for several months in the freezer.

- Dressed salads wilt quickly, so it's best to consume them the next day.
- Dishes with cooked seafood should be eaten within three days.
- Opened containers of nuts can be stored at room temperature for about two weeks. If keeping longer, it's best to freeze them.
- Whole grains can be stored at room temperature for up to a month. If keeping longer, it's best to freeze them.
- If reheating food in a microwave, be sure to use microwavable containers.
- Allow frozen food to thaw for several hours or overnight in the refrigerator before reheating in the microwave.
- If reheating on the stove top or in the oven, try to begin with fully thawed food. If food is still partially frozen, start at low heat until the food has thawed.

Once food has been reheated, it's best to not reheat it again; the quality of food usually decreases each time it's reheated.

Living Free of Chronic Inflammation

While this is essentially a cookbook, it's worth mentioning that inflammation can be exacerbated by everyday behaviors that may seem unrelated to food. Focus on the following tips, even one at a time, to build a strong foundation for your anti-inflammatory lifestyle.

SLEEP FOR AT LEAST 7 HOURS. Getting enough sleep reduces stress hormones and makes healthy choices easier. Include sleep as part of your planning and goal setting, and consider tracking the time you go to bed and wake up each day.

DRINK MORE WATER. This is not news, but it can't be emphasized enough. Water flushes out toxins and keeps the cells that hold us together healthy. It doesn't have to be the old "eight 8-ounce glasses a water per day." With more than 90 percent water content, watermelon, cantaloupe, grapefruit, and strawberries can help boost your intake. Carry a reusable water bottle with you, and commit to drink and refill it several times a day. Try add-ins like herbs and fruit to boost the flavor and health benefits (see Own Your Water, page 19). The best evidence that you're hydrating enough is that your urine is generally pale yellow.

BREATHE DEEPLY. Chronic stress puts cortisol levels into overdrive and increases inflammation. When you feel overwhelmed with tension, take a few deep breaths and remind yourself of your bigger goals. This will help de-escalate your feelings in the experience, even if you can't fix what's causing it.

INCLUDE EVERYONE. If you're the family-designated cook and there are multiple dietary needs to meet in your family, like vegan, paleo, or food allergies, use your own diet as the foundation, then consider how you can incorporate others' needs into what you are cooking.

GIVE YOURSELF SOME LEEWAY. When there's a special event on the calendar, lay out a strong foundation of healthy eating as you lead up to the big day. The day of, start off right with a breakfast from this book, and eat a nutritious snack before the big event so you're not hungry when you arrive. Once you're there, relax and enjoy! Give yourself permission to enjoy a few bites of your favorite special occasion treats as you focus on the folks, rather than the food. You can return to a more structured approach the following day, confident that you are creating sustainable real-life patterns that will endure.

GO ORGANIC. While the most important dietary change you can make is to eat more fresh fruits and vegetables, selecting organic produce when possible helps minimize exposure to potentially inflammatory pesticide residue. To get the biggest bang for your organic buck, consider the produce you consume most frequently or use a resource such as the Environmental Working Group's lists, The Dirty Dozen and the Clean Fifteen (see Appendix B, page 146).

CLEAN UP YOUR CLEANERS. Household products are one area where you can take a proactive stance to limit exposure to environmental toxins—and save money doing it. Buying or making your own natural cleaners, such as those that harness the cleansing power of vinegar or baking soda, ensures that what you spray in your home environment supports you in reducing inflammation. To learn more about the best products for your household, visit the Environmental Working Group's website at ewg.org.

CALL THE DOCTOR. If you haven't already, it's a good idea to see your health care provider before beginning any major dietary change. They can confirm that you're on the right track, and they might also measure blood levels that are indicative of inflammation. When you follow up after adopting anti-inflammatory eating principles, it can be reinforcing to see how those

tests results have improved! If you experience symptoms during your transition, like stomach pain, skin rashes, diarrhea, or other significant discomfort, be sure to see a doctor to rule out any underlying issues and find out how to proceed more comfortably.

BUST A MOVE. Find physical activities you enjoy and can stick with. Breaking a sweat helps you manage stress, maintain healthy weight, and increase energy. You don't have to become a marathon runner; research consistently shows that a regular walking routine is one of the most powerful ways to reduce disease risk and safeguard well-being.

QUIT SMOKING. Chronic exposure to cigarette smoke is linked with increased inflammatory cytokines and airway inflammation. Get help to ditch the habit, whether it's using a patch, joining a support group, or quitting with a friend. Mindfulness can help with cessation, as you can learn to take a few deep breaths and check in kindly with yourself when you're stressed, rather than reach immediately for a smoke.

We've discussed the ideal diet and explored behaviors that help ensure optimum health. You now have a range of ideas for how you can prepare for and build a long-term anti-inflammatory lifestyle. Which of these ideas inspire you? Begin with those that will build up your positive mindset as you get ready to start the anti-inflammatory diet—it's coming next!

PART TWO

Weekly Meal Plans with Recipes

Now that you've learned about the anti-inflammatory diet, let's put these ideas into practice. To help guide you, we've put together two weekly meal plans that are designed to be easy, convenient, and affordable. Most recipes yield two servings. Some of the recipes serve four to six people, but as part of the meal plan, they're intended to provide leftovers so you can reuse them for multiple meals. You'll come to love the resourceful "cook once, eat twice (or thrice!)" principle. As you become more comfortable with this plan, you can begin expanding your anti-inflammatory repertoire with the recipes in part 3 of this book.

The first step of starting any new diet is planning out your meals. Since we've already laid it out for you, spend a few minutes reviewing the weekly meal plans. The first day of each meal plan requires the most cooking, so you may want to start it on the day you're least busy, such as a day off from work.

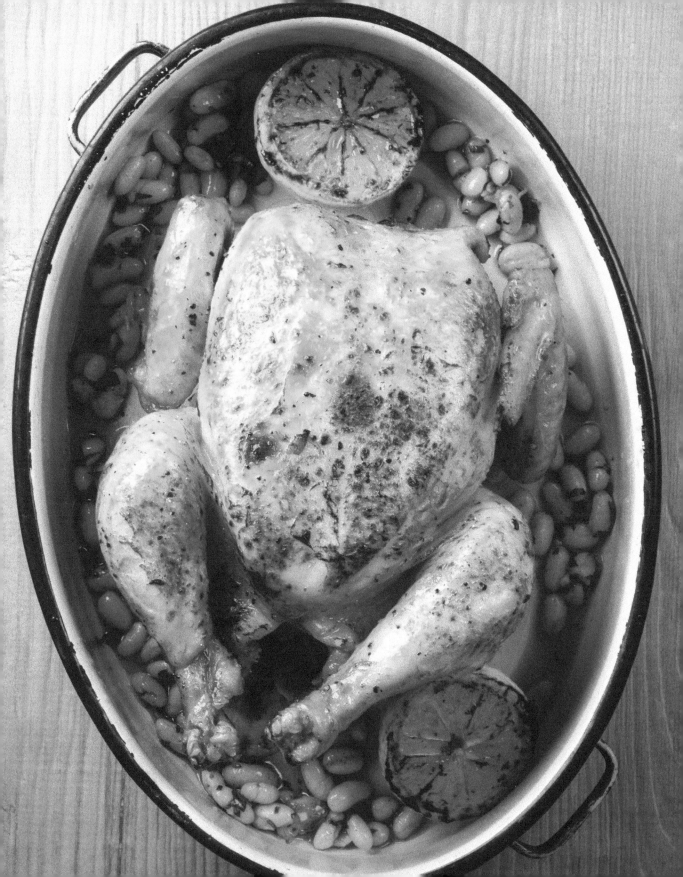

CHAPTER THREE

Week 1 Meal Plan and Recipes

This meal plan calls for bulk cooking on one day to give you meal options that last throughout the week. The menu is designed for two people; however, the recipes typically serve four to six, providing enough leftovers for an additional meal. We've included a breakfast, lunch, and dinner menu for Monday to Friday, and a brunch, snack, and dinner menu for Saturday and Sunday.

The recipes you'll need for this week's meal plan are arranged in meal groups, so all the breakfast recipes appear first, followed by the lunch recipes, then dinner, with the sides and snacks at the end.

Week 1 Meal Plan

M

BREAKFAST
- Sweet Potato Frittata* (page 45)

LUNCH
- Lentil-Beet Salad* (page 47)

DINNER
- Roast Chicken with Lemon and White Beans* (page 50)
- Roasted–Butternut Squash Mash* (page 57)

T

BREAKFAST
- Banana-Oat Muffins* (page 44)

LUNCH
- Leftover Roast Chicken with Lemon and White Beans

DINNER
- Brown Rice Bowl* (page 51)

W

BREAKFAST
- Greek Yogurt with Granola and Berries

LUNCH
- Miso Soup* (page 48)
- Leftover Brown Rice Bowl

DINNER
- Basic Baked Salmon* (page 52)
- Leftover Lentil-Beet Salad

TH

BREAKFAST
- Leftover Banana-Oat Muffins

LUNCH
- Vibrant Salmon Salad (page 49) (using leftover Basic Baked Salmon)

DINNER
- One-Pot Mushroom Pasta* (page 53)

F

BREAKFAST
- Greek Yogurt with Granola and Berries

LUNCH
- Leftover One-Pot Mushroom Pasta

DINNER
- Leftover Miso Soup
- Chopped Chicken and Apple Salad* (page 54)

SAT

BRUNCH
- Leftover Sweet Potato Frittata
- Melon Slices
- Lulu's Iced Coffee* (page 59)

SNACK
- Vegetable Sticks with Black Bean Dip* (page 60)

DINNER
- Chickpea and Kale Salad (page 55)

SUN

BRUNCH
- Coconut Pancakes* (page 46) with Greek Yogurt and Berries

SNACK
- Leftover Vegetable Sticks with Black Bean Dip

DINNER
- Balsamic-Glazed Chicken (page 56)
- Steamed Green Beans
- Rosemary Wild Rice* (page 58)

These dishes will be used later in the meal plan as leftovers, so you may want to make extra.

Shopping List

You'll need the following ingredients to prepare the recipes for this weekly meal plan. If you need ingredient substitutions due to food allergies, just check the recipes for substitution suggestions and revise the shopping list to suit your needs. If you wish, compare the ingredients against the Optional Weekly Prep Guide (page 43) to see if there are certain ingredients you want to buy pre-washed, already shredded, frozen, and so on.

CANNED AND BOTTLED ITEMS

* Black beans (1 [15-ounce] can)
* Broth, vegetable (8 cups)
* Broth, chicken (½ cup)
* Chickpeas (1 [15-ounce] can)
* Coconut or almond milk, unsweetened (3 cups)
* Lentils (2 [15-ounce] cans)
* Red wine, dry (¼ cup)
* White beans (1 [15-ounce] can)
* White wine, dry (½ cup)

DAIRY, MEAT/POULTRY, AND FISH

* Chicken, boneless, skinless breasts (6)
* Chicken, whole (1)
* Eggs, large (18)
* Greek yogurt, plain (6 cups)
* Salmon, boneless fillets (8 [3 to 4 ounces each])

PANTRY ITEMS

* Almond oil (optional)
* Apple cider vinegar
* Baking powder
* Baking soda
* Balsamic vinegar
* Chipotle powder
* Coconut oil (optional)
* Coffee
* Coriander, ground
* Cumin, ground
* Dijon mustard
* Honey
* Olive oil, extra-virgin
* Paprika
* Peppercorns, black
* Salt
* Turmeric, ground
* Vanilla extract
* White miso paste

OTHER

* Brown rice (2 cups uncooked)
* Cashews, raw (½ cup, optional)
* Coconut flour (1 cup)
* Granola
* Oat flour (1½ cups)
* Oats, quick-cooking (1 cup)
* Rigatoni (1 [12-ounce] package, gluten-free if necessary)
* Tofu, firm (½ cup)
* Walnuts (½ cup, optional)
* Wild rice (1 cup)

PRODUCE

- Apples, green (2 large)
- Avocados (2)
- Bananas (3 large)
- Beets, cooked (5)
- Berries (1 or 2 pints)
- Butternut squash (3 cups cubed)
- Carrot (2)
- Celery (1)
- Cilantro (1 bunch)
- Cucumber (1)
- Dill (1 bunch)
- Fennel bulbs (2)
- Garlic (1 head)
- Ginger root (1 small piece)
- Green beans (1 pound fresh or 1 [12-ounce] package frozen)
- Kale (1 large bunch)
- Lemons (6)
- Lettuce, romaine (1 heart)
- Lime (1)
- Melon (1 small)
- Mushrooms (2 cups)
- Onion, yellow (1)
- Onions, red (3 small)
- Potato, sweet (1 large)
- Rosemary (1 bunch)
- Scallions (1 bunch)
- Shallots (3)
- Spinach, baby (6 [6-ounce] bags)
- Tarragon (1 bunch)
- Thyme (1 bunch)
- Turmeric root (1 small piece)
- Additional vegetable sticks for snacking (cucumber, red bell peppers, etc.)

Recipes

BREAKFAST

- Banana-Oat Muffins
- Sweet Potato Frittata
- Coconut Pancakes

LUNCH

- Lentil-Beet Salad
- Miso Soup
- Vibrant Salmon Salad

DINNER

- Roast Chicken with Lemon and White Beans
- Brown Rice Bowl
- Basic Baked Salmon
- One-Pot Mushroom Pasta
- Chopped Chicken and Apple Salad
- Chickpea and Kale Salad
- Balsamic-Glazed Chicken

SIDE DISHES

- Roasted–Butternut Squash Mash
- Rosemary Wild Rice

SNACKS

- Lulu's Iced Coffee
- Vegetable Sticks with Black Bean Dip

Optional Weekly Prep Guide

One way to streamline meal preparation is to prep your ingredients in advance, just like on cooking shows. Some people find it helpful to batch-prep ingredients early in the week so they can cook recipes more quickly during busy weeknights. Others like to prep ingredients as they go. However you choose to do it, as the week progresses, you'll need to prep the following ingredients as directed. We've also noted a couple of recipes that are easy to make ahead and save time later in the week. Do what works for you!

WASH AND CUT

* Green beans: trim (or use frozen green beans)
* Kale: remove thick stems
* Beets: slice
* Scallions: chop
* Red onion: thinly slice 1, chop the rest

* Yellow onion: chop
* Celery: chop ½ cup, cut the rest into sticks
* Fennel: slice
* Shallots: chop
* Garlic: slice 1 clove, chop 4 cloves

COOK AND STORE

* Brown rice: 4 cups cooked
* Chicken: 2 cooked boneless, skinless chicken breasts
* Sweet Potato Frittata (page 45)
* Banana-Oat Muffins (page 44)

MAKE AHEAD

* Lemony Mustard Dressing (page 142)
* Ginger-Turmeric Dressing (page 141)

Breakfast in a muffin is so convenient, and a great way to use up bananas past their prime. This recipe gets its sweetness from the bananas, so there's no added sugar. If you prefer a sweeter muffin, you can add ½ cup sliced pitted dates, or ⅓ cup raw honey or maple syrup. Meal Plan Tip: Freeze half of the muffins for next week.

BANANA-OAT MUFFINS

MAKES 12 MUFFINS / PREP TIME: 15 MINUTES / COOK TIME: 25 MINUTES

SOY-FREE

GLUTEN-FREE

NUT-FREE

VEGETARIAN

MEDITERRANEAN

1½ cups oat flour (certified gluten-free, if necessary)

1 cup quick-cooking oats (certified gluten-free, if necessary)

1 tablespoon baking powder

½ teaspoon baking soda

½ teaspoon salt

3 large bananas, mashed

2 large eggs, slightly beaten

⅓ cup extra-virgin olive oil or almond oil

1. Preheat the oven to 375°F. Line a muffin pan with paper baking cups.
2. In a medium bowl, whisk together the oat flour, oats, baking powder, baking soda, and salt.
3. Add the mashed bananas, eggs, and oil and mix well. The batter will be thick.
4. Spoon the batter evenly into the prepared muffin cups.
5. Bake until the tops spring back when lightly touched, 20 to 25 minutes. Serve warm or at room temperature.

RECIPE TIP: If you aren't restricted, toasted walnuts, almonds, or hazelnuts are a good addition to this recipe. Whole-grain baked goods dry out more quickly than conventional baked goods, so it's best to store these in an airtight container in the freezer.

SUBSTITUTION TIP: To make this recipe vegan, replace each egg with 1 tablespoon ground flaxseed mixed with 3 tablespoons water.

NUTRITIONAL INFORMATION PER SERVING (1 muffin): Calories: 170; Total Fat: 9g; Total Carbohydrates: 21g; Sugar: 4g; Fiber: 2g; Protein: 4g; Sodium: 260mg

This is the easiest one-pan frittata out there! Sweet potatoes and red onions cook up in a cast-iron skillet until tender; then you simply add the beaten eggs and cook until firm. If you don't have a cast iron-skillet, you can use a pie plate.

SWEET POTATO FRITTATA

SERVES 4 / PREP TIME: 15 MINUTES / COOK TIME: 30 MINUTES

SOY-FREE

GLUTEN-FREE

NUT-FREE

VEGETARIAN

PALEO

MEDITERRANEAN

1 tablespoon extra-virgin olive oil, plus more for brushing

1 large sweet potato, peeled and cut into 1-inch pieces

1 small red onion, chopped

1 teaspoon salt

¼ teaspoon freshly ground black pepper

1 teaspoon chopped fresh thyme leaves

8 large eggs, well beaten

1. Preheat the oven to 375°F. Brush a cast-iron skillet with a little olive oil.
2. Toss together the sweet potato and onion in the skillet. Drizzle with 1 tablespoon olive oil and add the salt and pepper. Bake until the potato is tender, 10 to 15 minutes.
3. Remove the skillet from the oven and sprinkle the thyme over the vegetables. Carefully pour the eggs over the vegetables and return the skillet to the oven. Bake until the eggs are firm and jiggle only slightly if you shake the skillet, about 15 minutes.
4. Let cool for at least 5 minutes before cutting into wedges and serving.

RECIPE TIP: Once cool, the frittata can be stored in the refrigerator for up to a week. And it's not just for breakfast—enjoy a slice of frittata for lunch or dinner!

SUBSTITUTION TIP: This technique can be used to make any frittata. Zucchini, leeks, and rosemary, or new potatoes, red bell peppers, and basil are a couple of good combinations to try.

NUTRITIONAL INFORMATION PER SERVING: Calories: 220; Total Fat: 14g; Total Carbohydrates: 9g; Sugar: 2g; Fiber: 1g; Protein: 15g; Sodium: 760mg

Coconut flour has become the mainstay of many gluten-free recipes. It thickens as the batter sits, so you may need to add more coconut milk while you're cooking the pancakes. Because the texture is a bit dry, these tasty pancakes are at their best topped with fresh berries and plain yogurt. Meal Plan Tip: Double the batter recipe so you can make waffles next week with the leftovers.

COCONUT PANCAKES

SERVES 4 / PREP TIME: 10 MINUTES / COOK TIME: ABOUT 5 MINUTES PER PANCAKE

SOY-FREE

GLUTEN-FREE

NUT-FREE

VEGETARIAN

PALEO

MEDITERRANEAN

½ cup coconut flour

½ teaspoon baking soda

¼ teaspoon salt

1 cup unsweetened coconut milk

4 large eggs, lightly beaten

½ teaspoon vanilla extract

3 tablespoons extra-virgin olive oil

1. In a medium bowl, whisk together the coconut flour, baking soda, and salt.
2. Add the coconut milk, eggs, and vanilla and stir until smooth. If the batter is too thick, thin with additional coconut milk or water.
3. Melt 1 tablespoon of the oil in a large skillet over medium heat.
4. Add the batter in ½-cup scoops and cook until golden brown on the bottom, about 3 minutes. Flip and cook for about 2 minutes more.
5. Stack the pancakes on a plate while cooking the remaining batter. Serve immediately.

RECIPE TIP: This batter can also be prepared as waffles. Instead of cooking on the stove top, pour about ⅔ cup batter onto a preheated waffle iron and cook according to the manufacturer's directions. This recipe will make about 4 waffles. Once cooled, refrigerate the waffles in an airtight container until ready to serve. Reheat in a toaster oven.

NUTRITIONAL INFORMATION PER SERVING (2 pancakes): Calories: 340, Total Fat: 29g; Total Carbohydrates: 10g; Sugar: 2g; Fiber: 5g; Protein: 10g; Sodium: 400mg

Cooked beets and canned lentils make quick work of this convenient salad. Some markets sell cooked beets in the produce department. You may also find cooked lentils in the produce department and in the canned food section. This salad can be dressed up or down depending on your sensitivities and preferences. Try it topped with toasted walnuts and crumbled feta cheese.

LENTIL-BEET SALAD

SERVES 4 / PREP TIME: 15 MINUTES

SOY-FREE

GLUTEN-FREE

NUT-FREE

VEGAN

MEDITERRANEAN

4 cups baby spinach

1 (15-ounce) can lentils, drained and rinsed

4 cooked peeled beets, cut into 8 pieces

1 small red onion, sliced

⅓ cup extra-virgin olive oil

1 tablespoon apple cider vinegar

1 teaspoon salt

¼ teaspoon freshly ground black pepper

1 teaspoon chopped fresh tarragon leaves (optional)

1. Arrange the spinach leaves on a serving platter or in a bowl.
2. Top with the lentils, beets, and red onion.
3. In a small bowl, whisk together the olive oil, cider vinegar, salt, and pepper.
4. Drizzle the salad with the dressing, top with the tarragon (if using), and serve.

INGREDIENT TIP: If you can't find roasted beets in your store, you can make them yourself. Preheat the oven to 375°F. Peel 3 large beets, cut into quarters, and place on a double thickness of aluminum foil. Drizzle the beets with olive oil and add salt and pepper. Wrap the beets in the foil, place on a rimmed baking sheet, and cook until tender, 30 to 40 minutes. Cool, then prepare the salad as directed.

NUTRITIONAL INFORMATION PER SERVING: Calories: 320; Total Fat: 18g; Total Carbohydrates: 29g; Sugar: 7g; Fiber: 10g; Protein: 11g; Sodium: 640mg

Miso is a fermented paste made from either soybeans or grains like barley; like other fermented products, miso aids in digestion. This soup is quick, easy, nourishing, and generally very restorative. Make this pick-me-up dish your own by adding whatever you like to the soup. In this recipe, it's a simple broth adorned with tofu and scallions.

MISO SOUP

SERVES 4 / PREP TIME: 10 MINUTES / COOK TIME: 5 MINUTES

GLUTEN-FREE

NUT-FREE

VEGAN

MEDITERRANEAN

4 cups vegetable broth

2 slices peeled ginger root

2 slices peeled turmeric root

1 garlic clove, lightly crushed

3 to 4 tablespoons white miso

½ cup cubed firm tofu

1 scallion, thinly sliced

1. Pour the vegetable broth into a large pot and add the ginger root, turmeric root, and garlic. Bring to a boil over medium-high heat. Reduce to a simmer and simmer for 5 minutes.
2. Using a slotted spoon, remove and discard the ginger root, turmeric root, and garlic.
3. Put the miso in a small bowl, add one ladleful of hot broth, and whisk until smooth. Stir the miso broth mixture back into the pot and mix well.
4. Divide the broth among four serving bowls.
5. Divide the tofu and scallion among the bowls, and serve.

INGREDIENT TIP: Learning about miso is akin to learning about wines. There are many varieties—white, yellow, or light brown miso is more delicate and sweet in flavor, and darker red miso has a stronger, robust flavor. Give them all a try to learn which variety you prefer. I recommend organic miso since soybeans are often cultivated with lots of pesticides. Miso paste lasts for a long time in the refrigerator. Since this recipe uses only a small amount of tofu, the remaining tofu can be frozen for another meal.

NUTRITIONAL INFORMATION PER SERVING: Calories: 40; Total Fat: 1g; Total Carbohydrates: 4g; Sugar: 1g; Fiber: 1g; Protein: 3g; Sodium: 530mg

This colorful, nutrient-packed recipe uses the rest of the Basic Baked Salmon (page 52) served for dinner this week. Make this salad using any greens or other vegetables you like—it's also delightful topped with Ginger-Turmeric Dressing (page 141) or Lemony Mustard Dressing (page 142). If salt is a health concern for you, use plain grilled salmon in this dish rather than the preseasoned fillets from the menu plan. This will lower the recipe's overall sodium content.

VIBRANT SALMON SALAD

SERVES 2 / PREP TIME: 15 MINUTES

SOY-FREE

GLUTEN-FREE

NUT-FREE

VEGETARIAN

PALEO

MEDITERRANEAN

3 cups baby spinach

½ cucumber, thinly sliced

1 small fennel bulb, trimmed and thinly sliced

2 leftover Basic Baked Salmon fillets (page 52), flaked

1 small ripe avocado, peeled, pitted, and sliced

¼ cup extra-virgin olive oil

2 tablespoons fresh lemon juice

1 teaspoon salt

¼ teaspoon freshly ground black pepper

1 teaspoon chopped fresh dill

1. Arrange the spinach on a serving platter or in a bowl.
2. Top with the cucumber, fennel, salmon, and avocado.
3. In a small bowl, whisk together the olive oil, lemon juice, salt, pepper, and dill, or shake in a small jar with a tight-fitting lid.
4. Pour the dressing over the salad, and serve.

SUBSTITUTION TIP: Did you eat all that yummy salmon the other night? If so, you can use canned salmon or tuna, or some smoked salmon for a twist. If using smoked salmon, plan on 1 to 2 ounces per person, since smoked salmon is richer than baked salmon. To make this recipe vegan, substitute a 15-ounce can of chickpeas or black beans, drained and rinsed, for the salmon.

NUTRITIONAL INFORMATION PER SERVING: Calories: 590; Total Fat: 48g; Total Carbohydrates: 20g; Sugar: 6g; Fiber: 10g; Protein: 23g; Sodium: 3060mg

You'll easily impress your guests with this hearty one-pot supper because it looks more complicated to make than it actually is. The chicken is roasted in a Dutch oven; then the beans are added near the end so they can soak up all the hearty flavors from the chicken.

ROAST CHICKEN WITH LEMON AND WHITE BEANS

SERVES 4 TO 6 / PREP TIME: 15 MINUTES / COOK TIME: 1 HOUR 45 MINUTES

SOY-FREE

GLUTEN-FREE

NUT-FREE

MEDITERRANEAN

1 tablespoon extra-virgin olive oil

1 (3½- to 4-pound) chicken

1 teaspoon salt

¼ teaspoon freshly ground black pepper

1 onion, sliced

2 garlic cloves, thinly sliced

½ cup chicken broth

½ cup dry white wine

1 (15-ounce) can white beans, drained and rinsed

2 tablespoons fresh lemon juice

1. Preheat the oven to 375°F.
2. Heat the olive oil in a large Dutch oven over high heat.
3. Pat the chicken dry with a paper towel and add the salt and pepper.
4. Place the chicken, breast-side down, in the Dutch oven and brown the skin for 4 to 5 minutes. Turn the chicken over and brown the back.
5. Scatter the onion and garlic slices around the chicken and add the broth and white wine. Cover the Dutch oven and bake for 1 hour.
6. Add the white beans and lemon juice, cover, and cook for an additional 30 minutes.
7. Uncover and let the chicken cool for 10 minutes before serving.

SUBSTITUTION TIP: This dish can be made with a roasted whole chicken from your local market. Simply combine all the ingredients in a Dutch oven, cover, and bake in a 350°F oven for 30 minutes just to heat everything through.

NUTRITIONAL INFORMATION PER SERVING (4 portions): Calories: 460; Total Fat: 12g; Total Carbohydrates: 27g; Sugar: 2g; Fiber: 6g; Protein: 57g; Sodium: 700mg

What could be cozier than a mound of vegetables and proteins over a bed of grains? Grain bowls are an excellent way to use up leftovers and provide a nutrient-dense meal. This recipe uses brown rice, often considered one of the most digestible grains. Serve this dish warm or at room temperature.

BROWN RICE BOWL

SERVES 4 / PREP TIME: 15 MINUTES

SOY-FREE

GLUTEN-FREE

NUT-FREE

VEGAN

MEDITERRANEAN

4 cups cooked brown rice

2 cups baby spinach

½ cucumber, thinly sliced

1 cooked peeled beet, sliced

½ thinly sliced carrot

½ small red onion, thinly sliced

1 cup canned lentils

1 ripe avocado, peeled, pitted, and sliced

½ cup raw cashews (optional)

¼ cup chopped fresh cilantro (optional)

½ cup Ginger-Turmeric Dressing (page 141)

1. Divide the rice among four bowls.
2. Scatter the spinach on top of the rice.
3. Top with the cucumber, beet, carrot, and red onion.
4. Add the lentils and avocado.
5. Sprinkle the cashews and/or cilantro over the top (if using).
6. Drizzle the dressing over each bowl, and serve.

RECIPE TIP: This recipe is a breeze since all the prep can be done ahead—all that remains is to assemble and serve. If serving this dish warm, it's best to reheat the rice first, before building the bowls, so the cucumbers and carrots stay crunchy and the avocado doesn't get warm.

NUTRITIONAL INFORMATION PER SERVING: Calories: 750; Total Fat: 47g; Total Carbohydrates: 72g; Sugar: 5g; Fiber: 12g; Protein: 16g; Sodium: 350mg

The moistness of salmon makes it an excellent fish for almost any preparation. This fish is simply prepared with salt, pepper, and lemon juice, then baked. Be sure to let it rest for 5 to 10 minutes after taking it out of the oven because it will continue to gently cook. Meal Plan Tip: Double the recipe; you'll use the other half for tomorrow's lunch.

BASIC BAKED SALMON

SERVES 4 / PREP TIME: 5 MINUTES / COOK TIME: 15 MINUTES

SOY-FREE

GLUTEN-FREE

NUT-FREE

PALEO

MEDITERRANEAN

Extra-virgin olive oil, for brushing the pan

4 (3- to 4-ounce) boneless salmon fillets

1 teaspoon salt

¼ teaspoon freshly ground black pepper

2 tablespoons fresh lemon juice

1. Preheat the oven to 375°F. Lightly brush a 9-inch square baking pan with oil.
2. Place the salmon in the pan. Add the salt and pepper, then drizzle with the lemon juice.
3. Bake until the fish is cooked through, 10 to 15 minutes.
4. Remove from the oven and let rest for 5 to 10 minutes before serving.

RECIPE TIP: Not sure if the salmon is done? There are two ways to tell. You can touch the salmon at the thickest part and see if it's firm—if it is, then it's done. You can also use a fork to gently pull apart one or two of the flakes of the fillets in the thickest part. If it's still bright pink inside, return it to the oven for a few more minutes.

NUTRITIONAL INFORMATION PER SERVING: Calories: 180, Total Fat: 11g;
Total Carbohydrates: <1g; Sugar: 0g; Fiber: 0g; Protein: 19g; Sodium: 630mg

As crazy as it sounds, in this recipe the pasta and sauce cook together. That way the pasta absorbs the mushroom juices, creating a really flavorful, satisfying dish—and with one less pot to worry about! A generous dusting of grated Parmesan cheese is the perfect way to finish off this dish.

ONE-POT MUSHROOM PASTA

SERVES 4 TO 6 / PREP TIME: 15 MINUTES / COOK TIME: 20 MINUTES

SOY-FREE

NUT-FREE

VEGAN

MEDITERRANEAN

2 tablespoons extra-virgin olive oil, plus more for drizzling

2 cups quartered button or cremini mushrooms

1 teaspoon salt

¼ teaspoon freshly ground pepper

¼ cup dry red wine

1 shallot, minced

1 garlic clove, minced

1 (12-ounce) package rigatoni

4 to 4½ cups water

1 teaspoon chopped fresh rosemary (optional)

1. Heat the olive oil in a Dutch oven over high heat. Once hot, add the mushrooms, salt, pepper, and red wine. Cook, stirring occasionally, until the mushrooms are cooked, about 5 minutes.
2. Add the shallot and garlic and stir to combine.
3. Add the rigatoni and 4 cups of water and bring to a boil. Reduce to a simmer, cover, and cook until the pasta is tender and most of the water is absorbed, 12 to 15 minutes.
4. If the mixture is too thick, add up to ½ cup more water. Transfer to a serving bowl, drizzle with olive oil, top with the rosemary (if using), and serve.

RECIPE TIP: This dish can be refrigerated for up to a week, then reheated and served.

SUBSTITUTION TIP: If you're avoiding gluten, you can substitute gluten-free pasta.

NUTRITIONAL INFORMATION PER SERVING (4 portions): Calories: 390; Total Fat: 9g; Total Carbohydrates: 67g; Sugar: 3g; Fiber: 4g; Protein: 11g; Sodium: 580mg

This light, refreshing meal is easy to throw together with items prepped on your prep day. The lemony mustard dressing complements the sweetness of the apples, and the toasted walnuts are more than delicious—they contain an amino acid that supports blood vessel health. Delicious and nutritious!

CHOPPED CHICKEN AND APPLE SALAD

SERVES 2 / PREP TIME: 15 MINUTES

SOY-FREE

GLUTEN-FREE

MEDITERRANEAN

2 cooked boneless, skinless chicken breasts, cut into ½-inch cubes

½ cup chopped celery

1 large green apple, cored and coarsely chopped

1 romaine lettuce heart, chopped

3 scallions, chopped

½ cup canned chickpeas

½ cup Lemony Mustard Dressing (page 142)

½ cup chopped toasted walnuts (optional)

1. Combine the chicken, celery, apple, romaine, scallions, and chickpeas in a large bowl.
2. Add the dressing and toss to mix.
3. Divide the salad among four serving bowls, top with the toasted walnuts (if using), and serve.

RECIPE TIP: Except for the green apple, all the ingredients for this salad can be prepped ahead and kept in separate containers in the fridge until ready to assemble. The walnuts can be stored at room temperature.

INGREDIENT TIP: If you weren't able to cook the chicken ahead of time, you can easily make this salad using a roast chicken from your local market.

NUTRITIONAL INFORMATION PER SERVING: Calories: 860; Total Fat: 61g; Total Carbohydrates: 39g; Sugar: 20g; Fiber: 12g; Protein: 45g; Sodium: 590mg

This colorful salad, ready in minutes, features chickpeas sautéed in olive oil with garlic and then poured over kale to slightly wilt the kale. Chopped fennel and red onion add crunch and flavor, and the lemon juice brightens it all up. If you like, you can dot this salad with goat cheese before serving.

CHICKPEA AND KALE SALAD

SERVES 2 / PREP TIME: 15 MINUTES / COOK TIME: 5 MINUTES

SOY-FREE

GLUTEN-FREE

NUT-FREE

VEGAN

MEDITERRANEAN

¼ cup extra-virgin olive oil

1 cup canned chickpeas, drained and rinsed

1 garlic clove, thinly sliced

½ teaspoon ground cumin

1 large bunch kale, stems removed and leaves torn into bite-size pieces

½ cup chopped fennel

¼ cup chopped red onion

1 teaspoon salt

½ teaspoon paprika

¼ cup fresh lemon juice

1. In a large skillet, heat the olive oil over high heat.
2. Add the chickpeas, garlic, and cumin and sauté for 5 minutes.
3. Put the kale in a large bowl. Pour the hot chickpeas over the kale, tossing to slightly wilt the kale.
4. Add the fennel and red onion. Add the salt and paprika, drizzle with the lemon juice, and serve.

SUBSTITUTION TIP: If kale isn't your thing, this salad is just as good made with spinach or Swiss chard.

NUTRITIONAL INFORMATION PER SERVING: Calories: 470; Total Fat: 29g; Total Carbohydrates: 46g; Sugar: 5g; Fiber: 11g; Protein: 11g; Sodium: 1,090mg

Balsamic vinegar and honey pack a flavorful punch in this recipe. The chicken comes out moist and tender, with a sweet-tart essence infused by the vinegar and honey. Serve this chicken with steamed green beans and Rosemary Wild Rice (page 58). Meal Plan Tip: Save half of the chicken for lunch in week 2.

BALSAMIC-GLAZED CHICKEN

SERVES 4 / PREP TIME: 10 MINUTES / COOK TIME: 20 MINUTES

SOY-FREE

GLUTEN-FREE

NUT-FREE

MEDITERRANEAN

¼ cup balsamic vinegar

2 tablespoons honey

1 shallot, minced

1 teaspoon salt

4 boneless, skinless chicken breasts

1. Preheat the oven to 350°F.
2. Combine the balsamic vinegar, honey, shallot, and salt in a 9-by-13-inch baking pan and stir until the honey has dissolved.
3. Add the chicken, turning to coat.
4. Bake until the chicken is cooked through, about 20 minutes.
5. Let rest for 5 minutes before serving.

SUBSTITUTION TIP: You can make this recipe using pork chops instead of chicken. If using bone-in pork chops, allow an additional 5 minutes of cooking time.

NUTRITIONAL INFORMATION PER SERVING: Calories: 230; Total Fat: 4g; Total Carbohydrates: 12g; Sugar: 11g; Fiber: 0g; Protein: 35g; Sodium: 670mg

To mash or not to mash? They're irresistible mashed, but you can also enjoy these roasted vegetables as is or as part of a salad. Either way, carrots and apples add a nice sweetness to this comfort food. Leftovers can be added to the Roasted–Butternut Squash Soup with Sage and Pomegranate Seeds (page 100).

ROASTED–BUTTERNUT SQUASH MASH

SERVES 4 / PREP TIME: 10 MINUTES / COOK TIME: 30 MINUTES

SOY-FREE

GLUTEN-FREE

NUT-FREE

VEGETARIAN

PALEO

MEDITERRANEAN

3 cups cubed butternut squash

1 cup coarsely chopped carrot

1 large green apple, peeled, cored, and chopped

3 tablespoons extra-virgin olive oil

1 teaspoon salt

¼ teaspoon freshly ground black pepper

½ cup unsweetened almond milk

1. Preheat the oven to 375°F.
2. Combine the squash, carrot, and apple in a large bowl. Add the oil, salt, and pepper and toss to mix well.
3. Transfer the vegetables to a rimmed baking sheet and roast until the vegetables are tender and lightly browned, 20 to 30 minutes.
4. Return the vegetables to the bowl.
5. Using a potato masher, mash the vegetables, then add the milk and stir until mostly smooth. (The mixture will be slightly lumpy.) Serve immediately.

SUBSTITUTION TIP: For a twist, try this recipe using sweet potatoes instead of butternut squash.

NUTRITIONAL INFORMATION PER SERVING: Calories: 170; Total Fat: 11g; Total Carbohydrates: 20g; Sugar: 7g; Fiber: 4g; Protein: 2g; Sodium: 630mg

Wild rice isn't a rice at all, but rather a grass that was originally grown in the Great Lakes region of North America. Wild rice is high in protein and has a nutty, chewy flavor. It doesn't absorb liquid easily, so it needs a long, slow cook to soften and release its flavor. It can also be expensive, so if you wish, you can make this recipe with brown rice instead. Meal Plan Tip: Save half of this recipe for week 2.

ROSEMARY WILD RICE

SERVES 4 / PREP TIME: 10 MINUTES / COOK TIME: 45 MINUTES

SOY-FREE

GLUTEN-FREE

NUT-FREE

VEGAN

PALEO

MEDITERRANEAN

1 cup wild rice

3½ cups vegetable broth

1 tablespoon extra-virgin olive oil

1 teaspoon salt

¼ teaspoon freshly ground black pepper

1 teaspoon chopped fresh rosemary (optional)

1. Rinse the wild rice in a fine-mesh strainer and drain well. Transfer to a medium pot.
2. Add the broth, olive oil, salt, and pepper.
3. Bring to a boil over a high heat, then reduce to a simmer. Partially cover the pot to allow steam to escape and cook for 35 to 45 minutes. The rice is done when some of the strands break open.
4. Drain any additional liquid, then add the rosemary (if using), fluff the rice with a fork, and serve.

SUBSTITUTION TIP: If you decide to use brown rice, use 1 cup rice to 2½ cups water or vegetable broth. Also, reduce the cooking time to 30 to 40 minutes.

RECIPE TIP: Any leftover rice can be stored in an airtight container in the refrigerator for up to 5 days, or frozen for longer.

NUTRITIONAL INFORMATION PER SERVING: Calories: 190; Total Fat: 4g; Total Carbohydrates: 33g; Sugar: 2g; Fiber: 3g; Protein: 6g; Sodium: 710mg

Here's an iced coffee recipe that will surely satisfy. Most iced coffees are loaded with sweeteners, and often laden with fat. This recipe has no sugar, and if you don't take your coffee black, you can lighten it with coconut or almond milk. The vanilla stands in nicely for the sugar, but if you really miss having a sweetener, try adding a small amount of maple syrup!

LULU'S ICED COFFEE

SERVES 2 / PREP TIME: 5 MINUTES

SOY-FREE

GLUTEN-FREE

NUT-FREE

VEGAN

PALEO

MEDITERRANEAN

2 cups cold brewed coffee

½ cup unsweetened almond milk

¼ teaspoon vanilla extract

1 cup ice

1. Combine the coffee, milk, and vanilla in a pitcher.
2. Divide the ice between two tall glasses.
3. Pour the iced coffee over the ice and serve.

RECIPE TIP: To boost the flavor profile, add a cinnamon stick or some whole cloves. Let the spices steep in the iced coffee for at least 15 minutes before removing and serving. For a different texture, instead of pouring the coffee over ice, blend all the ingredients in a blender for a frozen iced coffee.

NUTRITIONAL INFORMATION PER SERVING: Calories: 10; Total Fat: <1g; Total Carbohydrates: <1g; Sugar: 0g; Fiber: <1g; Protein: 1g; Sodium: 50mg

Chipotle powder, lime juice, and cilantro give this dip an unmistakable Latin flavor. Canned beans make it a breeze to throw together—it's likely to become your new go-to party dip. Enjoy with sticks of carrots, celery, bell peppers, cucumbers, or other vegetables.

VEGETABLE STICKS WITH BLACK BEAN DIP

SERVES 4 TO 6 / PREP TIME: 15 MINUTES

SOY-FREE

GLUTEN-FREE

NUT-FREE

VEGAN

MEDITERRANEAN

1 (15-ounce) can black beans, drained and rinsed

2 scallions, chopped

1 tablespoon chopped fresh cilantro

2 tablespoons extra-virgin olive oil

2 tablespoons fresh lime juice

1 teaspoon chipotle powder

1 teaspoon salt

½ teaspoon ground cumin

1 cup carrot sticks, for serving

1 cup celery sticks, for serving

1. Combine all the ingredients except for the vegetable sticks in a medium bowl and toss to mix.
2. Using a potato masher, mash the ingredients until the mixture has a texture that's slightly smooth but still lumpy.
3. Serve with the vegetable sticks for dipping.

RECIPE TIP: This dip also makes a great spread for lettuce wraps. Store leftovers in an airtight contained in the refrigerator for up to a week.

SUBSTITUTION TIP: Beans are loaded with protein, fiber, and minerals. Any bean can be substituted for black beans in this recipe. Canned, drained white beans, garbanzo beans, and lentils are all good options. Or use an equal amount of thawed fava or lima beans for a springtime dip.

NUTRITIONAL INFORMATION PER SERVING (4 portions): Calories: 170; Total Fat: 7g; Total Carbohydrates: 20g; Sugar: 3g; Fiber: 7g; Protein: 6g; Sodium: 630mg

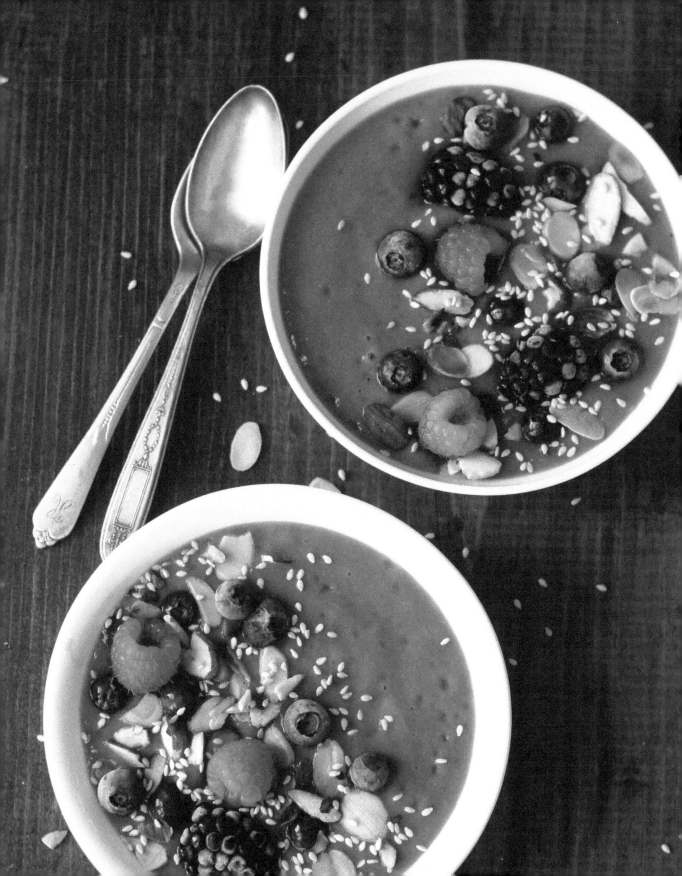

CHAPTER FOUR

Week 2 Meal Plan and Recipes

Now that you've gotten the hang of things, let's explore our next meal plan. Like the week 1 meal plan, this menu is designed for bulk cooking on one day to give you meal options that last throughout the week. The menu is designed for two people; however, the recipes typically serve four to six, yielding enough leftovers for an additional meal. We've provided a breakfast, lunch, and dinner menu for Monday through Friday, and a brunch, snack, and dinner menu on the weekend.

Just like last week, the recipes you'll need for this week's meal plan are arranged in meal groups, so all the breakfast recipes appear first, followed by the lunch recipes, then dinner, with the sides and snacks at the end.

Week 2 Meal Plan

M	**BREAKFAST** • Leftover Coconut Pancakes (made into waffles) with Yogurt and Berries	**LUNCH** • Leftover Balsamic-Glazed Chicken, Steamed Green Beans, and Rosemary Wild Rice	**DINNER** • Fennel Baked Salmon* (page 74) • Roasted Sweet Potatoes* (page 80) • Zucchini and Red Onion Salad with Olives* (page 81)
T	**BREAKFAST** • Overnight Oats (page 68)	**LUNCH** • Sweet Potato and Salmon Salad (page 71) (using leftover Fennel Baked Salmon, Roasted Sweet Potatoes, and Zucchini and Red Onion Salad with Olives)	**DINNER** • Chickpea and Feta Casserole* (page 75)
W	**BREAKFAST** • Mashed Avocado Spread on Bread (gluten-free if necessary) with Sea Salt	**LUNCH** • Turkey Taco Soup* (page 72)	**DINNER** • Chicken and Broccoli Stir-Fry* (page 76)
TH	**BREAKFAST** • Leftover Coconut Waffles with Yogurt and Berries	**LUNCH** • Leftover Chickpea and Feta Casserole	**DINNER** • Leftover Turkey Taco Soup
F	**BREAKFAST** • Mashed Avocado Spread on Bread (gluten-free if necessary) with Sea Salt	**LUNCH** • Leftover Chicken and Broccoli Stir-Fry	**DINNER** • Pan-Seared Pork Loin* (page 77) • Roasted Fingerling Potatoes (page 82) • Sautéed Spinach (page 83)
SAT	**BRUNCH** • Green Smoothie Bowl (page 69)	**SNACK** • Smoked Salmon and Chive Deviled Eggs* (page 84)	**DINNER** • Spinach and Pork Salad (using Leftover Pan-Seared Pork Loin)
SUN	**BRUNCH** • Avocado and Mango Salad (page 70) • Leftover Smoked Salmon and Chive Deviled Eggs	**SNACK** • Turmeric-Almond Smoothie (page 85)	**DINNER** • Mushroom-Shallot Risotto (page 79)

These dishes will be used later in the meal plan as leftovers, so you may want to make extra.

WEEK 2
Shopping List

You'll need the following ingredients to prepare the recipes for this weekly meal plan. If you need ingredient substitutions due to food allergies, just check the recipes for substitution suggestions and revise the shopping list to suit your needs. In addition, you can check against the Optional Weekly Prep Guide (page 66) to see if there are certain ingredients you want to buy prewashed, already shredded, frozen, and so on.

CANNED AND BOTTLED ITEMS

- Almond butter (optional)
- Coconut, almond, or soy milk, unsweetened (2¼ cups)
- Black beans (1 [15-ounce] can)
- Broth, chicken or vegetable (7 cups)
- Chickpeas (1 [15-ounce] can)
- Fire-roasted tomatoes (1 [14.5-ounce] can, optional)
- Red wine, dry (½ cup)
- White wine, dry (½ cup)

DAIRY, MEAT/POULTRY, AND FISH

- Cheese, feta (½ cup)
- Cheese, goat (4 ounces)
- Cheese, Parmesan (½ cup grated, optional)
- Chicken, boneless, skinless thighs (1 pound)
- Eggs, large (10)
- Greek yogurt, plain (4 cups)
- Pork loin roast, boneless (3 to 4 pounds)
- Salmon, boneless (4 [3- to 4-ounce] fillets)
- Salmon, smoked (4 ounces)
- Tofu, silken (8 ounces)
- Turkey, ground (1 pound)

PANTRY ITEMS

- Chipotle powder
- Coriander, ground
- Cumin, ground
- Dijon mustard
- Ginger, ground
- Honey
- Maple syrup
- Oil, coconut
- Oil, toasted sesame (optional)
- Olive oil, extra-virgin
- Oregano, dried
- Peppercorns, black
- Red pepper flakes
- Rosemary, dried
- Salt
- Toasted coconut (optional)
- Turmeric, ground
- Vanilla extract

OTHER

- Almonds (optional)
- Bread (gluten-free if necessary)
- Chia seeds
- Granola (1 package, preferably gluten-free and no added sugar)
- Oats
- Olives, green, pitted, sliced (½ cup)
- Pecans (optional)
- Rice, Arborio
- Sesame seeds

FROZEN

- Corn (1 [10-ounce] package)
- Spinach (1 [10-ounce] package)

PRODUCE

* Apples, green (2)
* Arugula (2 cups)
* Avocados (4)
* Banana (1)
* Bell pepper, red (1)
* Berries (1 to 2 pints)
* Broccoli (1 bunch)
* Chives (1 bunch, optional)
* Cilantro (1 bunch, optional)
* Fennel (1 bulb)
* Fingerling potatoes (1½ pounds)
* Garlic (1 head)
* Ginger root (1 small piece)
* Lemon (1)
* Lettuce, romaine (1 heart)
* Lime (1)
* Mango (1)
* Mushrooms (10 large)
* Onions, red (2)
* Onion, yellow (1)
* Parsley (1 bunch, optional)
* Pear (1)
* Potatoes, sweet (4 large)
* Radishes (2)
* Scallions (1 bunch)
* Shallot (1)
* Spinach (3 [6-ounce] bags)
* Zucchini (4)

Optional Weekly Prep Guide

As mentioned last week, some people find it helpful to batch-prep ingredients early in the week to save them time during busy weeknights. Others like to prep as they go. At some point, you'll need to prep the following ingredients as directed. We've also noted a couple of recipes that are easy to make ahead and save time later in the week.

WASH AND CUT

* Fennel: thinly slice
* Red onion: thinly slice
* Yellow onion: chop
* Zucchini: chop 1, thinly slice 2
* Red bell pepper: slice
* Radishes: slice and store in water until ready to use

COOK AND STORE

* Eggs: 6 hardboiled
* Turkey Taco Soup (page 72)

MAKE AHEAD

* Lemony Mustard Dressing (page 142)
* Ginger-Turmeric Dressing (page 141)

WEEK 2
Recipes

BREAKFAST

* Overnight Oats
* Green Smoothie Bowl
* Avocado and Mango Salad

LUNCH

* Sweet Potato and Salmon Salad
* Turkey Taco Soup

DINNER

* Fennel Baked Salmon
* Chickpea and Feta Casserole
* Chicken and Broccoli Stir-Fry
* Pan-Seared Pork Loin
* Spinach and Pork Salad
* Mushroom-Shallot Risotto

SIDES AND SNACKS

* Roasted Sweet Potatoes
* Zucchini and Red Onion Salad with Olives
* Roasted Fingerling Potatoes
* Sautéed Spinach
* Smoked Salmon and Chive Deviled Eggs
* Turmeric-Almond Smoothie

In a perfect world we'd wake up to long-simmered steel cut oats, but who has the time? This breakfast recipe is assembled the night before, and overnight the oats soften and the mixture thickens and becomes chewy and delicious. You can pop it in the microwave for a minute before adding your toppings, if you like. The optional chia seeds are packed with fiber, protein, and omega-3s—add them to just about anything for a nutritional boost!

OVERNIGHT OATS

SERVES 2 / PREP TIME: 10 MINUTES

SOY-FREE

GLUTEN-FREE

NUT-FREE

VEGAN

MEDITERRANEAN

1 cup oats (certified gluten-free if necessary)

1¾ cups unsweetened almond milk

2 tablespoons maple syrup

1 tablespoon chia seeds (optional)

¼ teaspoon vanilla extract

Optional Toppings

¼ cup almond butter

1 cup mixed berries

½ cup Greek yogurt

1 tablespoon toasted almonds

1 tablespoon toasted coconut

1. Combine the oats, milk, maple syrup, chia seeds (if using), and vanilla in a jar with a tight-fitting lid and shake well.
2. Refrigerate overnight.
3. When ready to serve, divide between two serving bowls and add your favorite toppings.

SUBSTITUTION TIP: If you're not vegan, you can make overnight oats using honey instead of maple syrup, and yogurt in place of coconut or almond milk.

NUTRITIONAL INFORMATION PER SERVING: Calories: 270; Total Fat: 8g; Total Carbohydrates: 50g; Sugar: 13g; Fiber: 7g; Protein: 8g; Sodium: 160mg

This smoothie bowl is a highly nutritious cold soup embellished with fruits and nuts. Thicker than a regular smoothie, it requires a spoon to enjoy. You can also add granola or toasted grains for a twist on the standard yogurt, fruit, and granola breakfast.

GREEN SMOOTHIE BOWL

SERVES 2 / PREP TIME: 15 MINUTES

SOY-FREE

GLUTEN-FREE

NUT-FREE

VEGAN

PALEO

MEDITERRANEAN

3 cups packed baby spinach

1 green apple, cored

1 small ripe banana

½ ripe avocado

1 tablespoon maple syrup

½ cup mixed berries

¼ cup toasted slivered almonds (optional)

1 teaspoon sesame seeds

1. Combine the spinach, apple, banana, avocado, and maple syrup in a blender and blend until smooth. The mixture should be thick.
2. Divide the mixture between two bowls. Top with the berries, almonds (if using), and sesame seeds, and serve.

SUBSTITUTION TIP: If you're not sensitive to soy, you can add ½ cup silken tofu to this recipe. Pitted dates are a great natural alternative to the maple syrup, if you prefer.

NUTRITIONAL INFORMATION PER SERVING (including almonds): Calories: 280; Total Fat: 14g; Total Carbohydrates: 38g; Sugar: 21g; Fiber: 9g; Protein: 6g; Sodium: 40mg

Avocados are loaded with healthy fats, potassium, and vitamins, plus a touch of protein. Mangos are packed with antioxidants and vitamins, and their sweet-tart flavor pairs beautifully with the buttery avocado. Ginger-Turmeric Dressing tops this wonderful anti-inflammatory breakfast salad.

AVOCADO AND MANGO SALAD

SERVES 2 / PREP TIME: 10 MINUTES

SOY-FREE

GLUTEN-FREE

NUT-FREE

VEGAN

PALEO

MEDITERRANEAN

1 romaine lettuce heart, chopped

1 large mango, sliced

1 avocado, peeled, pitted, and sliced

1 tablespoon chopped fresh chives

¼ cup Ginger-Turmeric Dressing (page 141)

¼ cup toasted almonds (optional)

1. Divide the lettuce between two serving bowls.
2. Arrange the mango and avocado slices on top of the lettuce.
3. Sprinkle the chives over the salads.
4. Drizzle the salads with the dressing, top with the almonds (if using), and serve.

INGREDIENT TIP: Mangos have a large pit that runs vertically down the middle of the fruit. To cut this fruit, hold the mango on its side on a cutting board. Run a knife through the mango along the side of the pit, cutting as close to the pit as you can—you won't be able to see the pit, so you'll have to feel it with your knife. You should now have half of a mango without a pit. Repeat the process to remove the second half of the mango from the pit. Then, without cutting through the skin, cut the flesh into slices, then turn the skin inside out—the slices will pop out. You can nudge them out with your fingers or a paring knife. You can store peeled mango for up to 4 days in a tightly covered container in the refrigerator.

NUTRITIONAL INFORMATION PER SERVING (including almonds): Calories: 500; Total Fat: 39g; Total Carbohydrates: 40g; Sugar: 26g; Fiber: 13g; Protein: 8g; Sodium: 310mg

Monday night dinner becomes Tuesday lunch in this delicious smorgas-bord salad. Fennel Baked Salmon, Roasted Sweet Potatoes, and Zucchini and Red Onion Salad with Olives are combined with fresh greens—it couldn't be easier. If salt is a health concern for you, use plain grilled salmon in this dish rather than the preseasoned fillets from the menu plan. This will lower the recipe's overall sodium content.

SWEET POTATO AND SALMON SALAD

SERVES 2 / PREP TIME: 10 MINUTES

SOY-FREE

GLUTEN-FREE

NUT-FREE

PALEO

MEDITERRANEAN

2 cups arugula or other greens

2 leftover Fennel Baked Salmon fillets (page 74), flaked

1 leftover Roasted Sweet Potato (page 80), cut in wedges

1 cup leftover Zucchini and Red Onion Salad with Olives (page 81)

¼ cup Lemony Mustard Dressing (page 142)

1. Combine the arugula, salmon, sweet potato wedges, and zucchini salad in a medium bowl.
2. Pour the dressing over and toss to mix, then serve.

RECIPE TIP: To make this even easier, assemble this salad on Monday evening while you put the dinner leftovers away; just keep the arugula and dressing on the side until you're ready to serve.

NUTRITIONAL INFORMATION PER SERVING: Calories: 570; Total Fat: 42g; · Total Carbohydrates: 22g; Sugar: 19g; Fiber: 5g; Protein: 22g; Sodium: 1,650mg

This hearty, health-supportive soup can be put together in minutes. Feel free to add or remove ingredients as you like; if you have a sensitivity to corn, omit it, or if you don't like beans, you can omit those as well. But if you can have it all, this robust soup will likely become a family favorite.

TURKEY TACO SOUP

SERVES 4 TO 6 / PREP TIME: 15 MINUTES / COOK TIME: 20 MINUTES

SOY-FREE

GLUTEN-FREE

NUT-FREE

MEDITERRANEAN

1 tablespoon extra-virgin olive oil

1 pound ground turkey

1 zucchini, sliced

2 garlic cloves, minced

1 teaspoon salt

1 teaspoon chipotle powder

½ teaspoon ground cumin

¼ teaspoon freshly ground black pepper

1 (15-ounce) can black beans, drained and rinsed

1 (14.5-ounce) can fire-roasted tomatoes with their juice (optional)

1 cup frozen corn (optional)

4 cups chicken or vegetable broth

Optional Toppings

Greek yogurt

Chopped scallions

Chopped fresh cilantro

1. In a Dutch oven, heat the oil over high heat.
2. Add the ground turkey and cook, stirring frequently, until browned, about 5 minutes.
3. Add the zucchini, garlic, salt, chipotle powder, cumin, and pepper and sauté until tender, about 5 minutes.
4. Add the black beans, fire-roasted tomatoes (if using), corn (if using), and broth.

5. Bring to a boil, then reduce to a simmer and simmer to heat through and combine the flavors, about 10 minutes.
6. Ladle into bowls and serve, passing around toppings if desired.

RECIPE TIP: Once cooled, this soup can be frozen in quart jars to have on hand for a quick meal.

SUBSTITUTION TIP: To make this soup vegan, substitute a 15-ounce can of kidney beans, drained and rinsed, for the turkey, and use vegetable broth. To make it paleo, omit the corn and the beans, double the zucchini, and add 2 cups cauliflower florets.

NUTRITIONAL INFORMATION PER SERVING (soup only): Calories: 370; Total Fat: 14g; Total Carbohydrates: 33g; Sugar: 2g; Fiber: 10g; Protein: 29g; Sodium: 1,020mg

Salmon is loaded with omega-3s, and fennel is a good digestive aid. If you like fennel, you'll enjoy how its anise flavor permeates the salmon. This recipe uses a power beverage—a bit of wine—to bake the fish in; if you are avoiding wine, substitute vegetable broth or water instead. Since the oven is already on to bake the salmon, I often pop in some roasted vegetables or potatoes to go along with this dish.

FENNEL BAKED SALMON

SERVES 4 / PREP TIME: 10 MINUTES / COOK TIME: 20 MINUTES

SOY-FREE

GLUTEN-FREE

NUT-FREE

PALEO

MEDITERRANEAN

1 tablespoon extra-virgin olive oil

1 fennel bulb, thinly sliced

½ small red onion, thinly sliced

4 (3- to 4-ounce) boneless salmon fillets

1 teaspoon salt

¼ teaspoon freshly ground black pepper

½ cup dry white wine

1. Preheat the oven to 375°F. Brush a 9-inch square baking pan with the olive oil.
2. Scatter the fennel and red onion slices in the bottom of the pan.
3. Add the salmon fillets and the salt and pepper. Pour in the wine.
4. Bake until the salmon is firm to the touch and flakes with a fork, about 20 minutes.
5. Let the salmon rest for 5 minutes before serving.

RECIPE TIP: This weekly plan calls for saving half of this dish to use as part of your lunch salad the next day. If you don't use it for the salad, you can store cooked salmon in the refrigerator for up to 3 days.

NUTRITIONAL INFORMATION PER SERVING: Calories: 250; Total Fat: 14g; Total Carbohydrates: 6g; Sugar: 3g; Fiber: 2g; Protein: 20g; Sodium: 670mg

This is a solid meal in an easy casserole! The feta, cumin, and oregano give this recipe a decidedly Mediterranean flavor, and the chickpeas and zucchini provide protein and a satisfying texture. I like to serve this filling dish with a simple salad of spinach seasoned with lemon juice and sea salt.

CHICKPEA AND FETA CASSEROLE

SERVES 6 TO 8 / PREP TIME: 15 MINUTES / COOK TIME: 30 MINUTES

SOY-FREE

GLUTEN-FREE

NUT-FREE

VEGETARIAN

MEDITERRANEAN

2 tablespoons extra-virgin olive oil, plus more for brushing

1 large onion, chopped

1 zucchini, chopped

2 garlic cloves, chopped

1 (15-ounce) can chickpeas, drained and rinsed

½ cup crumbled feta cheese

1 teaspoon dried oregano

½ teaspoon ground cumin

½ teaspoon salt

¼ teaspoon freshly ground black pepper

4 large eggs, lightly beaten

1. Preheat the oven to 350°F. Brush a 9-by-13-inch baking pan with olive oil.
2. In a large skillet, heat 2 tablespoons of olive oil over high heat.
3. Add the onion, zucchini, and garlic and sauté until the vegetables begin to brown, about 5 minutes.
4. Transfer the cooked vegetables to a large bowl and add the chickpeas.
5. Using a potato masher, slightly mash the chickpeas and the vegetables.
6. Add the feta, oregano, cumin, salt, pepper, and eggs, and mix well.
7. Spoon the mixture into the prepared pan, smooth the top, and bake until firm, about 20 minutes.
8. Let cool for 5 to 10 minutes before serving.

RECIPE TIP: Once cooled, this casserole can be cut into squares and individually wrapped to take to work or have on hand for an easy meal. Store leftovers in the refrigerator for up to 5 days.

NUTRITIONAL INFORMATION PER SERVING (6 portions): Calories: 210; Total Fat: 12g; Total Carbohydrates: 16g; Sugar: 4g; Fiber: 4g; Protein: 10g; Sodium: 480mg

Stir-fry is the quintessential one-pot meal, and you can really have fun with this cooking style! If you don't want to take the time to prep broccoli for this tasty recipe, you can substitute spinach. Use two 5-ounce bags of baby spinach instead of the 2 cups of broccoli florets. That may seem like a lot, but spinach cooks down to nothing.

CHICKEN AND BROCCOLI STIR-FRY

SERVES 4 TO 6 / PREP TIME: 15 MINUTES / COOK TIME: 15 MINUTES

SOY-FREE

GLUTEN-FREE

NUT-FREE

PALEO

MEDITERRANEAN

2 tablespoons coconut oil

1 pound boneless, skinless chicken thighs, cut into thin strips

2 cups broccoli florets

2 garlic cloves, thinly sliced

1 teaspoon minced fresh ginger root

1 teaspoon salt

¼ teaspoon red pepper flakes

¾ cup chicken broth

1 teaspoon toasted sesame oil (optional)

1 tablespoon sesame seeds (optional)

1. In a Dutch oven, heat the coconut oil over high heat.
2. Add the chicken and sauté until it starts to brown, 5 to 8 minutes.
3. Add the broccoli florets, garlic, ginger, salt, red pepper flakes, and broth.
4. Cover the pot, lower the heat to medium, and let the mixture steam until the broccoli turns bright green, about 5 minutes.
5. Remove from the heat, add the sesame oil and sesame seeds (if using), and serve.

RECIPE TIP: It's easy to prep this meal ahead of time for an easy last-minute meal. The chicken can be cut into strips, the broccoli cut into florets, and the garlic and ginger chopped and ready to go. Store the chicken and broccoli in separate containers. The garlic and ginger can be stored together. Keep all ingredients in the refrigerator until ready to cook.

NUTRITIONAL INFORMATION PER SERVING (4 portions): Calories: 250; Total Fat: 14g; Total Carbohydrates: 5g; Sugar: <1g; Fiber: 1g; Protein: 27g; Sodium: 810mg

Pork offers a nice break from chicken and seafood. Though this juicy meat lags behind chicken and beef when it comes to sustainable farming—that which protects the land, people, communities, and animal welfare—pork farmers are catching up. Buying pork from the farmers' market is one way to ensure you're getting sustainably raised pork. Try serving this with Roasted Fingerling Potatoes (page 82) and Sautéed Spinach (page 83).

PAN-SEARED PORK LOIN

SERVES 4 TO 6 / PREP TIME: 15 MINUTES / COOK TIME: 45 MINUTES

SOY-FREE

GLUTEN-FREE

NUT-FREE

PALEO

MEDITERRANEAN

1 cup water

1 (3- to 4-pound) boneless pork loin roast

2 tablespoons extra-virgin olive oil

1½ teaspoons salt

½ teaspoon freshly ground black pepper

1 teaspoon dried rosemary

1. Preheat the oven to 375°F. Pour the water into a 9-by-13-inch roasting pan.
2. Heat a large skillet over high heat.
3. Coat the roast with the olive oil and place it in the hot skillet. Brown on all sides, 2 to 3 minutes per side.
4. Transfer the browned roast to the roasting pan. Combine the salt, pepper, and rosemary in a small bowl and sprinkle the seasonings evenly over the meat.
5. Roast until a meat thermometer inserted in the center reads 150°F, 30 to 40 minutes.
6. Let the roast rest for about 10 minutes before serving.

RECIPE TIP: Searing the meat before roasting adds nice color and extra flavor to the roast while keeping the interior moist. You can use this same technique with beef or lamb.

NUTRITIONAL INFORMATION PER SERVING (4 portions using 3-pound roast): Calories: 490; Total Fat: 18g; Total Carbohydrates: 0g; Sugar: 0g; Fiber: 0g; Protein: 76g; Sodium: 1,040mg

To eat potatoes or not to eat potatoes, that is the paleo conundrum. Some people do and some don't; some eat only sweet potatoes. If you aren't eating potatoes, you can substitute roasted cauliflower for the potatoes. This salad uses the leftovers from last night's dinner, Pan-Seared Pork Loin and Roasted Fingerling Potatoes, served over a bed of crunchy uncooked spinach.

SPINACH AND PORK SALAD

SERVES 2 / PREP TIME: 15 MINUTES / COOK TIME: NONE

SOY-FREE

GLUTEN-FREE

NUT-FREE

MEDITERRANEAN

2 cups baby spinach

8 (½-inch-thick) slices leftover Pan-Seared Pork Loin (page 77)

4 leftover Roasted Fingerling Potatoes (page 82), cut in half lengthwise

1 green apple, cored and thinly sliced

½ red bell pepper, thinly sliced

¼ cup Ginger-Turmeric Dressing (page 141)

¼ cup toasted pecans, chopped (optional)

1. In a medium bowl, toss together the spinach, pork loin, potatoes, green apple, and red bell pepper.
2. Pour the dressing over and toss to combine.
3. Divide between two bowls, top with the pecans (if using), and serve.

RECIPE TIP: If you're making this salad the night before, combine all the ingredients except the dressing and the pecans, then add them right before serving.

NUTRITIONAL INFORMATION PER SERVING (including pecans): Calories: 590; Total Fat: 39g; Total Carbohydrates: 19g; Sugar: 8g; Fiber: 5g; Protein: 42g; Sodium: 900mg

Risotto is made with short-grained rice, typically Arborio rice from Italy. If you are unable to find Arborio rice, you can still make it with other short-grained rice, but be aware that it will probably cook faster. Risotto has an unfounded reputation for being difficult—the secret is simply to add the liquid slowly while stirring, which gives the rice a chance to absorb the liquid as it slowly cooks. The result is a creamy, slightly chewy rice.

MUSHROOM-SHALLOT RISOTTO

SERVES 4 TO 6 / PREP TIME: 15 MINUTES / COOK TIME: 20 TO 25 MINUTES

SOY-FREE

GLUTEN-FREE

NUT-FREE

VEGAN

MEDITERRANEAN

2 tablespoons extra-virgin olive oil

1 large shallot, thinly sliced

10 large button or cremini mushrooms, sliced

½ cup dry red wine

1 cup Arborio rice

1½ to 2 cups vegetable broth

½ cup grated Parmesan cheese (optional)

1 tablespoon chopped fresh parsley

1 teaspoon salt

¼ teaspoon freshly ground black pepper

1. Heat the olive oil in a large skillet over high heat. Add the shallot and sauté until softened, 3 to 5 minutes.
2. Add the mushrooms and red wine and simmer until all the wine has evaporated.
3. Add the rice and sauté for about 3 minutes to coat the rice with the flavors in the pan.
4. Add ½ cup of broth and cook and stir occasionally until the broth has been absorbed. Add another ½ cup of broth and repeat. Continue until the risotto is tender but not mushy, about 20 minutes.
5. Remove from the heat. Sprinkle with the Parmesan cheese (if using), parsley, salt, and pepper, and serve.

RECIPE TIP: For variety, some toasted walnuts are also delicious in this dish—just add them right before serving. Leftovers will keep for about a week in the refrigerator.

NUTRITIONAL INFORMATION PER SERVING (4 portions, includes Parmesan): Calories: 320; Total Fat: 11g; Total Carbohydrates: 829g; Sugar: 2g; Fiber: 2g; Protein: 10g; Sodium: 830mg

Think of these as oven fries. Sweet potato wedges are coated in an anti-inflammatory spice mix including turmeric, coriander, and ginger, and roasted until slightly brown—this also brings out their yummy sweetness.

ROASTED SWEET POTATOES

SERVES 4 TO 6 / PREP TIME: 15 MINUTES / COOK TIME: 20 MINUTES

SOY-FREE

GLUTEN-FREE

NUT-FREE

VEGAN

PALEO

MEDITERRANEAN

2 tablespoons extra-virgin olive oil or melted coconut oil, plus more to brush the pans

3 large sweet potatoes, scrubbed and cut into thin wedges

1 teaspoon salt

1 teaspoon ground turmeric

½ teaspoon ground coriander

¼ teaspoon ground ginger

¼ teaspoon chipotle powder

1 lime

1. Preheat the oven to 400°F. Brush two rimmed baking sheets with olive oil.
2. Put the sweet potato wedges in a large bowl. Add 2 tablespoons of olive oil and toss to coat the potatoes.
3. In a small bowl, mix the salt, turmeric, coriander, ginger, and chipotle powder. Sprinkle the spice mix over the potatoes, mixing well to coat evenly.
4. Arrange the sweet potato wedges in a single layer on the prepared baking sheets.
5. Bake until the sweet potatoes are tender in the middle and slightly browned and caramelized on the edges, about 20 minutes.
6. Remove from the oven, squeeze lime juice over the wedges, and serve.

RECIPE TIP: You can make a triple batch of this spice mix to keep on hand for use as a seasoning for chicken, fish, or zucchini.

NUTRITIONAL INFORMATION PER SERVING (4 portions): Calories: 150; Total Fat: 7g; Total Carbohydrates: 20g; Sugar: 4g; Fiber: 3g; Protein: 2g; Sodium: 640mg

This kind of salad typically uses cucumbers, but this recipe calls for raw zucchini instead. Gardeners, this is a terrific recipe for all that zucchini you don't know what to do with! Plus, you will have the unique opportunity to enjoy this salad when the zucchini is at its freshest.

ZUCCHINI AND RED ONION SALAD WITH OLIVES

SERVES 4 / PREP TIME: 15 MINUTES

SOY-FREE

GLUTEN-FREE

NUT-FREE

VEGAN

PALEO

MEDITERRANEAN

1 cup arugula

2 large zucchinis, thinly sliced

½ small red onion, thinly sliced

2 radishes, thinly sliced

½ cup pitted green olives, sliced

2 tablespoons extra-virgin olive oil

2 tablespoons fresh lemon juice

1 teaspoon salt

⅛ teaspoon red pepper flakes

1. In a medium bowl, combine the arugula, zucchini, red onion, radishes, and green olives.
2. Add the olive oil, lemon juice, salt, and red pepper flakes and toss to combine. Serve.

RECIPE TIP: If you have a spiralizer, you can make zucchini "noodles" instead of slices. This salad lends itself well to lots of additions—chickpeas, toasted walnuts, or goat cheese will all complement the flavors of this dish. Leftovers can be stored in the refrigerator for several days.

NUTRITIONAL INFORMATION PER SERVING: Calories: 120; Total Fat: 10g; Total Carbohydrates: 7g; Sugar: 4g; Fiber: 3g; Protein: 2g; Sodium: 870mg

Fingerling potatoes are so named because they are long, skinny potatoes that could resemble fingers of, well, an elf or gnome! These thin-skinned treats cook quickly and have a nice sweet flavor.

ROASTED FINGERLING POTATOES

SERVES 4 TO 6 / PREP TIME: 5 MINUTES / COOK TIME: 20 MINUTES

SOY-FREE

GLUTEN-FREE

NUT-FREE

VEGAN

MEDITERRANEAN

2 tablespoons extra-virgin olive oil, plus more to brush the baking sheet

1½ pounds fingerling potatoes, scrubbed

1 teaspoon salt

¼ teaspoon freshly ground black pepper

1 tablespoon chopped fresh parsley or chives (optional)

1. Preheat the oven to 400°F. Brush a rimmed baking sheet with oil.
2. Put the potatoes in a large bowl. Add 2 tablespoons of oil and toss to coat the potatoes.
3. Toss the potatoes with the salt and pepper.
4. Arrange the potatoes in a single layer on the prepared baking sheet.
5. Bake until the potatoes are tender in the middle and slightly browned, about 20 minutes.
6. Remove from the oven, sprinkle with the parsley or chives (if using), and serve.

RECIPE TIP: Roasted fingerling potatoes make excellent potato salad. Using a potato masher, lightly mash them with 1 teaspoon Dijon mustard and ½ cup plain yogurt for a quick side dish.

NUTRITIONAL INFORMATION PER SERVING (4 portions): Calories: 180; Total Fat: 7g; Total Carbohydrates: 27g; Sugar: 2g; Fiber: 4g; Protein: 3g; Sodium: 610mg

Frozen spinach? Sure, why not? Since spinach wilts when you cook it, it takes a *lot* of fresh spinach to yield enough sautéed spinach to feed four people. Buy frozen chopped spinach and allow it to thaw completely before cooking. It really tastes good, especially with the enhancements of lemon and garlic.

SAUTÉED SPINACH

SERVES 4 / PREP TIME: 5 MINUTES / COOK TIME: 5 MINUTES

SOY-FREE

GLUTEN-FREE

NUT-FREE

VEGAN

PALEO

MEDITERRANEAN

1 tablespoons extra-virgin olive oil

1 (10-ounce) package frozen chopped spinach, thawed and drained

1 garlic clove, minced

1 teaspoon salt

¼ teaspoon freshly ground black pepper

1 tablespoon fresh lemon juice

1. In a large skillet, heat the oil over high heat.
2. Add the spinach, garlic, salt, and pepper and sauté until the spinach is heated through, about 5 minutes.
3. Add the lemon juice, stir to combine, and serve.

RECIPE TIP: Leftovers make a great bed for fried eggs, guaranteeing a colorful and extra nutritious breakfast.

NUTRITIONAL INFORMATION PER SERVING: Calories: 50; Total Fat: 4g; Total Carbohydrates: 3g; Sugar: 0g; Fiber: 2g; Protein: 2g; Sodium: 630mg

Once you've enjoyed these deviled eggs for breakfast, you can snack on the leftovers later. This spin on the traditional deviled egg combines high-protein, filling goodness with the satisfying richness of smoked salmon.

SMOKED SALMON AND CHIVE DEVILED EGGS

SERVES 4 TO 6 / PREP TIME: 20 MINUTES / COOK TIME: 10 MINUTES

SOY-FREE

GLUTEN-FREE

NUT-FREE

MEDITERRANEAN

6 hardboiled eggs, peeled

4 ounces goat cheese, at room temperature

1 teaspoon Dijon mustard

½ teaspoon salt

⅛ teaspoon freshly ground black pepper

4 ounces smoked salmon, thinly sliced

1 tablespoon chopped fresh chives

1. Cut the hardboiled eggs in half lengthwise; then carefully remove the egg yolks and place in a small bowl.
2. Mash the egg yolks with the goat cheese, mustard, salt, and pepper.
3. Spoon the egg mixture back into the egg white halves. Top with the smoked salmon and chives and serve.

INGREDIENT TIP: If possible, buy organic, pastured eggs. They are more expensive than conventional eggs, but they are even more delicious. Better yet, purchase eggs from a farm or farmers' market.

NUTRITIONAL INFORMATION PER SERVING (6 portions): Calories: 150; Total Fat: 10g; Total Carbohydrates: 1g; Sugar: 0g; Fiber: 0g; Protein: 14g; Sodium: 510mg

Pears, spinach, and avocado are the base for this uber-anti-inflammatory drink. And if that's not enough, we've also added tofu for protein and turmeric to bring it all home. Turmeric comes from the ginger family. It's a little bitter on its own, but works well combined with the other ingredients in this recipe.

TURMERIC-ALMOND SMOOTHIE

SERVES 2 / PREP TIME: 10 MINUTES

GLUTEN-FREE

NUT-FREE

VEGAN

MEDITERRANEAN

1 pear, cored and quartered

2 cups baby spinach

¼ avocado

1 cup silken tofu

1 teaspoon ground turmeric or 1 thin slice peeled turmeric root

½ cup unsweetened almond milk

2 tablespoons honey (optional)

1 cup ice

In a blender, combine all the ingredients and blend until smooth. Divide between two glasses, and serve.

SUBSTITUTION TIP: If pears aren't in season, you can substitute an apple for similar flavor and nutritional rewards.

NUTRITIONAL INFORMATION PER SERVING (including honey): Calories: 270; Total Fat: 11g; Total Carbohydrates: 38g; Sugar: 27g; Fiber: 6g; Protein: 10g; Sodium: 80mg

PART THREE

Anti-Inflammatory Recipes for Life

Now that you have two weeks under your belt, are you ready to make anti-inflammatory eating a daily part of your life? In this section we have provided simple, five-ingredient recipes using whole foods for breakfast and brunch, vegetarian and vegan, fish and shellfish, poultry and meat, and anti-inflammatory snacks and desserts! Many of the recipes can be made ahead and stored in single-serving portions for quick weekday meals.

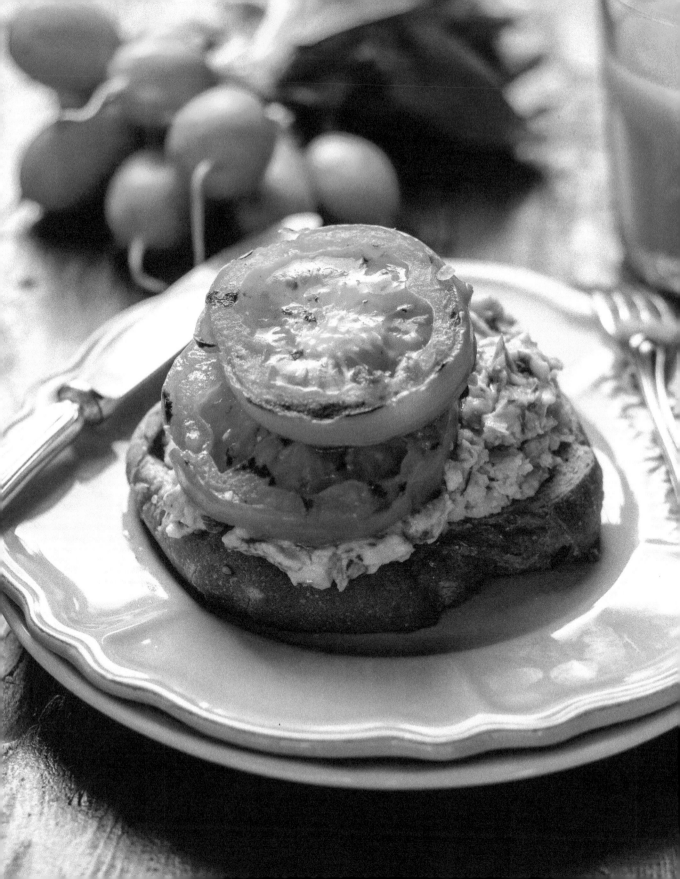

CHAPTER FIVE

Breakfast and Brunch

Opposite: Whole-Grain Toast with Chickpea Paste, Avocado, and Grilled Tomato, page 95

Green apples, spinach, maple syrup, and cinnamon are the core ingredients in this smoothie, making it taste like apple pie! Trust us: You won't really notice the spinach. For those who have trouble getting enough veggies, this is a good way to sneak some in.

GREEN ON GREEN SMOOTHIE

SERVES 1 / PREP TIME: 5 MINUTES

SOY-FREE

GLUTEN-FREE

NUT-FREE

VEGAN

PALEO

MEDITERRANEAN

1 cup packed baby spinach

½ green apple

1 tablespoon maple syrup

¼ teaspoon ground cinnamon

1 cup unsweetened almond milk

½ cup ice

In a blender, combine all the ingredients and blend until smooth. Serve.

RECIPE TIP: If you can eat nuts, a handful of raw pistachios blended with the rest of the ingredients adds a rich, buttery flavor and boosts protein.

NUTRITIONAL INFORMATION PER SERVING: Calories: 130; Total Fat: 4g; Total Carbohydrates: 23g; Sugar: 18g; Fiber: 3g; Protein: 2g; Sodium: 150mg

A little advance planning will yield a tempting breakfast you won't mind waking up early for. In this recipe, brown rice, milk, and vanilla get a long, slow cook in the slow cooker. You can serve this for Sunday brunch or make it the day before, then serve either cold or warm. Suggested toppings include fresh fruit, chopped apples, yogurt, or toasted nuts.

CINNAMON BROWN RICE PUDDING

SERVES 4 TO 6 / PREP TIME: 5 MINUTES / COOK TIME: 2½ TO 3 HOURS

SOY-FREE

GLUTEN-FREE

NUT-FREE

VEGAN

PALEO

MEDITERRANEAN

1 cup uncooked brown rice

3 cups unsweetened coconut or almond milk

¼ cup maple syrup

⅛ teaspoon salt

1 teaspoon vanilla extract

1 teaspoon ground cinnamon

1. In a slow cooker, combine the brown rice, milk, maple syrup, and salt and mix well.
2. Cover and cook on high until the rice is tender, 2½ to 3 hours.
3. Stir in the vanilla and cinnamon, and serve.

RECIPE TIP: To add sweetness, stir ½ cup raisins or dried cranberries into the rice before cooking it. Store leftovers in the refrigerator for up to a week, or freeze in convenient individual-size servings for longer.

NUTRITIONAL INFORMATION PER SERVING (4 portions): Calories: 250; Total Fat: 4g; Total Carbohydrates: 50g; Sugar: 12g; Fiber: 2g; Protein: 4g; Sodium: 720mg

Chia seeds are high in fiber and protein. When added to liquid, they soften and create a tapioca-like consistency. The oats provide more fiber and texture, and toasting them brings out their nutty flavor. You can dress up this treat any way you'd like—try adding sliced bananas, tropical fruits, and nuts.

CHIA PUDDING WITH OATS, STRAWBERRIES, AND KIWI

SERVES 2 / PREP TIME: 25 MINUTES

SOY-FREE

GLUTEN-FREE

VEGAN

MEDITERRANEAN

2 cups unsweetened almond milk

⅓ cup chia seeds

¼ cup maple syrup

½ teaspoon vanilla extract

½ cup toasted oats (see Tip)

4 large strawberries, sliced

1 kiwi, peeled and sliced

1. In a quart-size jar with a tight-fitting lid, combine the milk, chia seeds, maple syrup, and vanilla. Cover and shake well, then set aside for at least 15 minutes for the pudding to thicken. (This can even be done the night before and refrigerated overnight.)
2. Divide the pudding between two serving dishes, top with the toasted oats, strawberries, and kiwi, and serve.

RECIPE TIP: To add protein, you can make this with soy milk if you're not sensitive to soy. If you can't find toasted oats, they're a snap to make. Spread the oats on a rimmed baking sheet and place in a 375°F oven for 5 to 8 minutes, checking them after 5 minutes, and stirring the oats if necessary so they toast evenly. Once toasted, pour the oats into a bowl, since they will continue to cook if left on the hot baking sheet. Cool completely and store in an airtight container at room temperature—they will keep for several weeks.

NUTRITIONAL INFORMATION PER SERVING: Calories: 360; Total Fat: 11g; Total Carbohydrates: 60g; Sugar: 31g; Fiber: 12g; Protein: 8g; Sodium: 190mg

Rather than a grain, buckwheat is a plant that produces grain-like seeds. Buckwheat is rich in both manganese and magnesium, two minerals that improve cardiovascular health. In this crunchy snack recipe, maple syrup and pecans complement the nuttiness of the toasted buckwheat.

BUCKWHEAT GRANOLA

SERVES 6 / PREP TIME: 15 MINUTES / COOK TIME: 10 MINUTES

SOY-FREE

GLUTEN-FREE

VEGAN

PALEO

MEDITERRANEAN

3 cups buckwheat groats

½ cup coarsely chopped pecans

⅓ cup extra-virgin olive oil

¼ cup maple syrup

1 teaspoon vanilla extract

¼ teaspoon salt

1. Preheat the oven to 350°F.
2. In a medium bowl, combine the buckwheat, pecans, oil, maple syrup, vanilla, and salt. Mix well to evenly coat the buckwheat with the oil and maple syrup.
3. Spread the mixture on a rimmed baking sheet and place in the oven.
4. After 5 minutes, remove the baking sheet from the oven. Using a spatula, stir the mixture around so it will bake evenly. Return to the oven and bake until the granola is lightly toasted, about 5 minutes more.
5. Allow to cool completely before serving.

RECIPE TIP: If you'd like to add dried fruit to this granola, add it after baking and cooling the granola. Once cool, the granola can be stored at room temperature in an airtight container for up to 6 weeks.

NUTRITIONAL INFORMATION PER SERVING: Calories: 490; Total Fat: 21g; Total Carbohydrates: 71g; Sugar: 8g; Fiber: 9g; Protein: 11g; Sodium: 110mg

This "frittata" is an entirely different animal than the traditional egg version, using instead garbanzo bean (chickpea) flour, which adds a flavorful protein base. Get creative and add any vegetables you like to this recipe; mushrooms or red bell peppers are nice additions. If you're not vegan, feta cheese gives it a nice tang.

VEGAN "FRITTATA"

SERVES 6 / PREP TIME: 15 MINUTES / COOK TIME: 20 MINUTES

SOY-FREE

GLUTEN-FREE

NUT-FREE

VEGAN

MEDITERRANEAN

1½ cups garbanzo bean flour

1 teaspoon salt

1 teaspoon ground turmeric

½ teaspoon ground cumin

1 teaspoon chopped fresh sage

1½ cups water

2 tablespoons extra-virgin olive oil

1 zucchini, sliced

2 scallions, sliced

1. Preheat the oven to 350°F.
2. In a medium bowl, whisk together the garbanzo bean flour, salt, turmeric, cumin, and sage.
3. Slowly add the water, stirring constantly to prevent the batter from getting lumpy. Set aside.
4. In an oven-safe skillet, heat the oil over high heat. Sauté the zucchini until softened, 2 to 3 minutes. Stir in the scallions, then spoon the batter over the vegetables.
5. Place the skillet in the oven and bake until firm when jiggled slightly, 20 to 25 minutes.
6. Serve warm or at room temperature.

RECIPE TIP: Store in the refrigerator for a week, or consider freezing this dish in individual-size portions for handy grab-and-go work lunches.

NUTRITIONAL INFORMATION PER SERVING: Calories: 140; Total Fat: 6g; Total Carbohydrates: 15g; Sugar: 3g; Fiber: 3g; Protein: 6g; Sodium: 410mg

If you've never tried avocado toast, it's delicious—and this recipe takes it to a new level. This dish is tasty, filling, and satisfying and will hold you over until lunch.

WHOLE-GRAIN TOAST WITH CHICKPEA PASTE, AVOCADO, AND GRILLED TOMATO

SERVES 2 / PREP TIME: 15 MINUTES / COOK TIME: 5 MINUTES

SOY-FREE

NUT-FREE

VEGAN

MEDITERRANEAN

2 thick slices whole-grain bread

2 thick tomato slices

Extra-virgin olive oil, for brushing

¼ cup Chickpea Paste (page 131)

½ avocado, mashed

¼ teaspoon sea salt

Freshly ground black pepper, to taste

1. Toast the bread.
2. While the bread is toasting, heat a stove top grill or skillet over high heat.
3. Brush the tomato slices with olive oil. Grill the tomato slices until grill marks appear, 1 to 2 minutes per side. Transfer to a plate.
4. Once the bread has toasted, brush with olive oil. Divide the chickpea paste between the two slices of toast, spreading it evenly. Top with the mashed avocado, then place a slice of grilled tomato on top.
5. Sprinkle with sea salt and freshly ground pepper and serve immediately.

SUBSTITUTION TIP: Substitute gluten-free bread for the whole-grain bread if you're avoiding gluten. You can also substitute hummus for the chickpea paste if you like.

INGREDIENT TIP: Beefsteak tomatoes are preferred for this recipe, since they have dense flesh and almost no seeds. If beefsteaks aren't available, Roma tomatoes make a good substitute.

NUTRITIONAL INFORMATION PER SERVING: Calories: 220; Total Fat: 11g; Total Carbohydrates: 27g; Sugar: 2g; Fiber: 6g; Protein: 7g; Sodium: 680mg

Most of the breakfast sausages available at the grocery store are loaded with ingredients and stabilizers that don't support anti-inflammatory eating. This fast and easy recipe calls for ground chicken, but you can substitute ground turkey or pork or a combination of the two if you'd like to change it up. This recipe makes about 24 sausage patties. You can store them in the refrigerator or freezer and reheat whenever you crave a savory breakfast meat or snack.

SAVORY BREAKFAST SAUSAGE

SERVES 8 / PREP TIME: 15 MINUTES / COOK TIME: 15 MINUTES

SOY-FREE

GLUTEN-FREE

NUT-FREE

PALEO

MEDITERRANEAN

Extra-virgin olive oil, for brushing

1½ pounds ground chicken

2 scallions, sliced

1 tablespoon chopped fresh sage

1 teaspoon salt

¼ teaspoon freshly ground black pepper

½ teaspoon ground nutmeg

1 tablespoon Dijon mustard

1. Preheat the oven to 400°F. Brush a rimmed baking sheet with olive oil.
2. In a medium bowl, combine the chicken, scallions, sage, salt, pepper, nutmeg, and mustard. Mix gently until all the ingredients are evenly distributed throughout the chicken.
3. Using a 1-ounce ice cream scoop or spoon, scoop the mixture into 24 small mounds onto the prepared baking sheet.
4. With your fingers or the back of a spatula, gently flatten each mound into a patty shape.
5. Bake until firm to the touch, 10 to 15 minutes. Serve warm.

RECIPE TIP: It's easy to make this recipe into chicken sausage cups for brunch! Heat the oven to 375°F. Divide the uncooked mixture among 8 oiled muffin tins. Press the mixture into each tin so you've created a sausage crust. Gently crack an egg and place the egg in each sausage-lined tin. Place in the preheated oven and bake 15 minutes or until the egg is firm. Allow to cool about 5 minutes before removing from the tins and serving. To remove, gently run a knife along the edges of each tin to loosen and lift the sausage muffin out. Serve immediately. These are also great served room temperature for lunch with a side of greens!

INGREDIENT TIP: Try adding one small chopped apple for chicken-apple sausages, or change it up seasonally by substituting turkey for the chicken and adding 1/2 cup dried cranberries. Once cooled, the patties can be stored in an airtight container in the refrigerator for up to 3 days or frozen for longer.

NUTRITIONAL INFORMATION PER SERVING (3 patties): Calories: 130; Total Fat: 7g; Total Carbohydrates: <1g; Sugar: <1g; Fiber: <1g; Protein: 15g; Sodium: 390mg

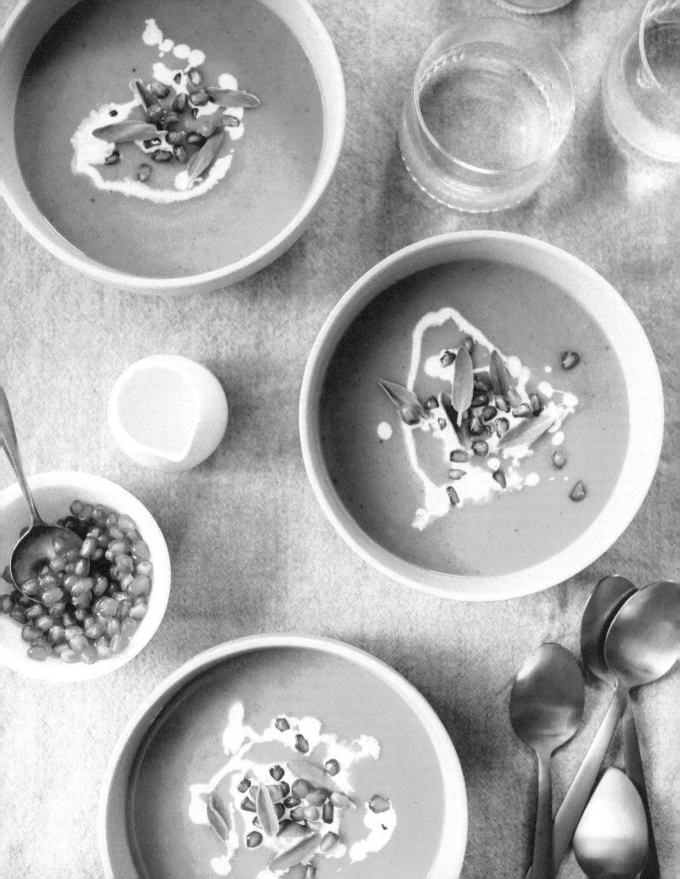

CHAPTER SIX

Vegetarian and Vegan

Opposite: Roasted–Butternut Squash Soup with Sage and Pomegranate Seeds, page 100

Either butternut squash or pumpkin purée can be substituted for the Roasted–Butternut Squash Mash in this recipe. Winter squash and sage are two flavors that go well together, and a topping of yogurt and pomegranate seeds rounds out this mouthwatering dish.

ROASTED–BUTTERNUT SQUASH SOUP WITH SAGE AND POMEGRANATE SEEDS

SERVES 4 / PREP TIME: 10 MINUTES / COOK TIME: 10 MINUTES

SOY-FREE

GLUTEN-FREE

NUT-FREE

PALEO

MEDITERRANEAN

2 tablespoons extra-virgin olive oil

2 shallots, finely chopped

1 garlic clove, minced

2 cups Roasted–Butternut Squash Mash (page 57)

2 cups vegetable or chicken broth

½ cup unsweetened coconut milk (optional)

1 teaspoon salt

¼ teaspoon freshly ground black pepper

8 fresh sage leaves

⅓ cup pomegranate seeds

¼ cup yogurt (optional)

1. In a Dutch oven, heat the oil over medium-high heat.
2. Add the shallots and garlic and sauté until softened, 3 to 5 minutes.
3. Add the butternut squash and broth and stir to combine.
4. Bring to a boil, reduce to a simmer, and cook for 3 to 5 minutes to heat through.
5. Add the coconut milk (if using) and season to taste with salt and pepper.
6. Garnish with the sage leaves, pomegranate seeds, and yogurt (if using) and serve.

RECIPE TIP: Store leftover soup in a covered container in the refrigerator for up to a week or in the freezer for several months.

INGREDIENT TIP: Many stores sell pomegranate seeds when in season. If you can't find pomegranate seeds, dried cranberries are a good substitute.

NUTRITIONAL INFORMATION PER SERVING (including coconut milk and yogurt): Calories: 200; Total Fat: 16g; Total Carbohydrates: 11g; Sugar: 4g; Fiber: 2g; Protein: 4g; Sodium: 820mg

Most stews take hours to cook, but this restorative dish, perfect for dinner or lunch, cooks up in a hurry. This plant-based recipe takes advantage of canned lentils and is loaded with nutritious anti-inflammatory power foods.

LENTIL STEW

SERVES 4 TO 6 / PREP TIME: 15 MINUTES / COOK TIME: 15 MINUTES

SOY-FREE

GLUTEN-FREE

NUT-FREE

VEGAN

MEDITERRANEAN

1 tablespoon extra-virgin olive oil

1 onion, chopped

3 carrots, peeled and sliced

8 Brussels sprouts, halved

1 large turnip, peeled, quartered, and sliced

1 garlic clove, sliced

6 cups vegetable broth

1 (15-ounce) can lentils, drained and rinsed

1 cup frozen corn

1 teaspoon salt

¼ teaspoon freshly ground black pepper

1 tablespoon chopped fresh parsley

1. In a Dutch oven, heat the oil over high heat.
2. Add the onion and sauté until softened, about 3 minutes.
3. Add the carrots, Brussels sprouts, turnip, and garlic and sauté for an additional 3 minutes.
4. Add the broth and bring to a boil. Reduce to a simmer and cook until the vegetables are tender, about 5 minutes.
5. Add the lentils, corn, salt, pepper, and parsley and cook for an additional minute to heat the lentils and corn. Serve hot.

RECIPE TIP: This soup is as versatile as it is simple. Feel free to use any kinds of beans or vegetables you have—it's a great way to use up leftover vegetables at the end of the week. Store in a covered container in the refrigerator for a week, or in the freezer for longer.

NUTRITIONAL INFORMATION PER SERVING (4 portions): Calories: 240; Total Fat: 4g; Total Carbohydrates: 42g; Sugar: 11g; Fiber: 12g; Protein: 10g; Sodium: 870mg

We're all used to white cauliflower, but other varieties include yellow cauliflower, purple cauliflower, and the greenish Roman cauliflower. A good produce market or farmers' market often sells all the varieties. However, if you can only find white, you'll still be delighted with the flavor when roasted—it just won't be as colorful.

ROASTED TRI-COLOR CAULIFLOWER

SERVES 4 TO 6 / PREP TIME: 10 MINUTES / COOK TIME: 20 MINUTES

SOY-FREE

GLUTEN-FREE

NUT-FREE

VEGAN

PALEO

MEDITERRANEAN

1½ cups white cauliflower florets

1½ cups purple cauliflower florets

1½ cups yellow cauliflower florets

3 tablespoons extra-virgin olive oil

¼ cup fresh lemon juice

1 teaspoon salt

¼ teaspoon freshly ground black pepper

1. Preheat the oven to 400°F.
2. In a large bowl, combine the cauliflower, olive oil, and lemon juice. Toss to coat well.
3. Spread the cauliflower on a rimmed baking sheet and add the salt and pepper.
4. Cover with aluminum foil and bake for 15 minutes. Remove the foil and continue to bake until the cauliflower starts to brown around the edges, about 5 minutes more.
5. Serve warm or at room temperature.

RECIPE TIP: Add a 15-ounce can of chickpeas or white beans, drained and rinsed, and 2 cups of cooked brown rice to turn this into a complete meal. You can also reuse any leftover cauliflower in salad recipes. Store in an airtight container in the refrigerator for up to a week.

NUTRITIONAL INFORMATION PER SERVING (4 portions): Calories: 120; Total Fat: 10g; Total Carbohydrates: 7g; Sugar: 3g; Fiber: 2g; Protein: 2g; Sodium: 620mg

Quinoa is a favorite superfood, and for good reason. This filling plant-based protein provides all nine essential amino acids that the body needs. Many markets carry cooked quinoa in the frozen foods aisle. This recipe utilizes already-cooked quinoa added to vegetables, making for a fast and easy skillet meal.

QUINOA WITH MIXED VEGETABLES

SERVES 4 TO 6 / PREP TIME: 10 MINUTES / COOK TIME: 15 MINUTES

SOY-FREE

GLUTEN-FREE

NUT-FREE

VEGAN

MEDITERRANEAN

3 tablespoons extra-virgin olive oil

1½ cups quartered Brussels sprouts

1 large zucchini, chopped

1 onion, chopped

3 garlic cloves, sliced

2½ cups cooked quinoa

1 cup vegetable broth or tomato sauce

1 tablespoon fresh lemon juice

1 teaspoon dried oregano

1 teaspoon salt

¼ teaspoon freshly ground black pepper

1. In a large skillet, heat the oil over high heat.
2. Add the Brussels sprouts, zucchini, onion, and garlic and sauté until the vegetables are tender, 5 to 7 minutes.
3. Add the quinoa and broth, cover, and cook for an additional 5 minutes.
4. Add the lemon juice, oregano, salt, and pepper and stir to fluff the quinoa.
5. Serve warm or at room temperature.

RECIPE TIP: Dish out some of these power leftovers when you need a pick-me-up between meals. Store in the refrigerator for up to 5 days, or freeze for longer.

NUTRITIONAL INFORMATION PER SERVING (4 portions): Calories: 270; Total Fat: 13g; Total Carbohydrates: 34g; Sugar: 5g; Fiber: 8g; Protein: 8g; Sodium: 640mg

This dish feels like something you could enjoy both at a summer picnic and on a cold night. Basil and garlic lend an Italian flavor to the pasta sauce used here, which is made of tofu and almond butter. Arugula adds a peppery flavor, and sliced asparagus delivers the crunch. This salad is equally delicious served slightly warm or cold.

GREEN PASTA SALAD

SERVES 4 TO 6 / PREP TIME: 15 MINUTES / COOK TIME: 15 MINUTES

GLUTEN-FREE

VEGAN

MEDITERRANEAN

1 (12-ounce) package gluten-free penne or fusilli

1 bunch asparagus, sliced on the diagonal into 1-inch pieces

1 tablespoon extra-virgin olive oil

1 cup Tofu-Basil Sauce (page 138)

2 cups arugula

2 scallions, sliced

1 teaspoon salt

¼ teaspoon freshly ground black pepper

1. Cook the pasta in a large pot of boiling water according to the package directions. Add the asparagus to the pot for the last 2 minutes of cooking time. Drain the pasta and asparagus in a colander, then return them to the pot.
2. Add the olive oil and sauce and stir to combine. Set aside to cool to room temperature.
3. Stir in the arugula, scallions, salt, and pepper and serve.

RECIPE TIP: You can make this dish ahead through step 2, then add the arugula and scallions right before serving. Store leftovers in a covered container in the refrigerator for up to 5 days.

NUTRITIONAL INFORMATION PER SERVING (4 portions): Calories: 450; Total Fat: 15g; Total Carbohydrates: 68g; Sugar: 3g; Fiber: 5g; Protein: 13g; Sodium: 290mg

The idea of making an omelet intimidates some people, but once you get the knack, they're really easy to make—and a great use of whatever scraps are left in your refrigerator. This omelet uses chives and parsley, but other good combinations are basil and garlic, or cilantro and scallion. Add some crumbled feta or a dollop of yogurt for added richness, if desired.

HERB OMELET

SERVES 2 / PREP TIME: 10 MINUTES / COOK TIME: 5 MINUTES

SOY-FREE

GLUTEN-FREE

NUT-FREE

VEGETARIAN

PALEO

MEDITERRANEAN

3 large eggs

1 tablespoon chopped fresh chives

1 tablespoon chopped fresh parsley

1 teaspoon ground turmeric

¼ teaspoon ground cumin

½ teaspoon salt

2 tablespoons extra-virgin olive, divided

1. In a medium bowl, whisk together the eggs, chives, parsley, turmeric, cumin, and salt.
2. In an omelet pan, heat 1 tablespoon of oil over medium-high heat.
3. Pour half of the egg mixture into the hot pan.
4. Reduce the heat to medium and let the eggs cook until the bottom starts to set.
5. Using a heat-proof spatula, gently move the eggs around the edges so the uncooked egg can spill over the sides of the cooked egg and set.
6. Continue to cook the omelet until just set, but still soft. Use the spatula to fold the omelet in half, then slide it out of the pan and onto a serving dish.
7. Repeat with the remaining egg mixture and 1 tablespoon of oil. Serve.

RECIPE TIP: For best results when preparing omelets, use a nonstick pan. The days of nonstick plastics are gone; you can now purchase reasonably priced nonstick pans made of ceramic materials that won't flake off (into your food!) over time.

NUTRITIONAL INFORMATION PER SERVING: Calories: 240; Total Fat: 21g; Total Carbohydrates: <1g; Sugar: <1g; Fiber: 0g; Protein: 11g; Sodium: 310mg

If you feel the need for a health boost, this dish will deliver. The vegetables are loaded with nutrients, and the curry powder contains many health-supportive properties. Feel free to change out the root vegetables with whatever vegetables look good at the market.

VEGETABLE CURRY

SERVES 4 TO 6 / PREP TIME: 15 MINUTES / COOK TIME: 15 MINUTES

SOY-FREE

GLUTEN-FREE

NUT-FREE

VEGAN

PALEO

MEDITERRANEAN

1 tablespoon coconut oil

1 onion, chopped

2 cups (½-inch) butternut squash cubes

1 large sweet potato, peeled and cut into ½-inch cubes

2 garlic cloves, sliced

1 (13.5-ounce) can coconut milk

2 cups vegetable broth

2 teaspoons curry powder

1 teaspoon salt

2 tablespoons chopped fresh cilantro

1. In a Dutch oven, heat the oil over high heat.
2. Add the onion and sauté until softened, about 3 minutes.
3. Add the butternut squash, sweet potato, and garlic and sauté for an additional 3 minutes.
4. Add the coconut milk, broth, curry powder, and salt and bring to a boil. Reduce to a simmer and cook until the vegetables are tender, about 5 minutes.
5. Top with the cilantro and serve.

INGREDIENT TIP: No curry powder? No problem—it's easy to make your own custom spice mix! It won't taste exactly like curry powder, but it will still be delicious. Combine 1 teaspoon ground turmeric, ½ teaspoon ground ginger, ½ teaspoon ground cumin, ½ teaspoon ground coriander, and ½ teaspoon ground cinnamon. Store any leftover spice mix in an airtight container at room temperature. This spice mix is also delicious sprinkled over baked sweet potatoes.

NUTRITIONAL INFORMATION PER SERVING (4 portions): Calories: 120; Total Fat: 5g; Total Carbohydrates: 20g; Sugar: 4g; Fiber: 3g; Protein: 2g; Sodium: 670mg

Whole-wheat pasta and walnuts are a classic Italian combination. Tucking Swiss chard into the recipe sneaks some vegetables in. If you're not vegan, enhance the yum factor with a dusting of freshly shaved Parmesan cheese.

WHOLE-WHEAT PENNE WITH WHITE BEANS, CHARD, AND WALNUTS

SERVES 4 TO 6 / PREP TIME: 10 MINUTES / COOK TIME: 18 MINUTES

SOY-FREE

VEGAN

MEDITERRANEAN

1 (12-ounce) package whole-wheat penne

2 tablespoons extra-virgin olive oil

1 bunch Swiss chard, cut into thin ribbons

1 garlic clove, sliced

1 teaspoon salt

⅛ teaspoon red pepper flakes

1 (15-ounce) can white beans, drained and rinsed

¼ cup chopped toasted walnuts (optional)

1. Cook the penne in a large pot of boiling water according to the package directions, then drain.
2. While the pasta is cooking, in a large skillet, heat the oil over high heat.
3. Add the chard, garlic, salt, and red pepper flakes and cook until the chard has wilted, about 3 minutes. Stir in the white beans until warm.
4. In a large serving bowl, toss together the penne and chard-bean mixture, mixing well. Sprinkle with the walnuts and serve.

RECIPE TIP: Try drizzling a bit more olive oil over this dish before serving. Store in a covered container in the refrigerator for up to 5 days.

SUBSTITUTION TIP: To make this gluten-free, use gluten-free pasta instead of whole-wheat penne.

NUTRITIONAL INFORMATION PER SERVING (4 portions including walnuts): Calories: 620; Total Fat: 14g; Total Carbohydrates: 101g; Sugar: 5g; Fiber: 17g; Protein: 25g; Sodium: 660mg

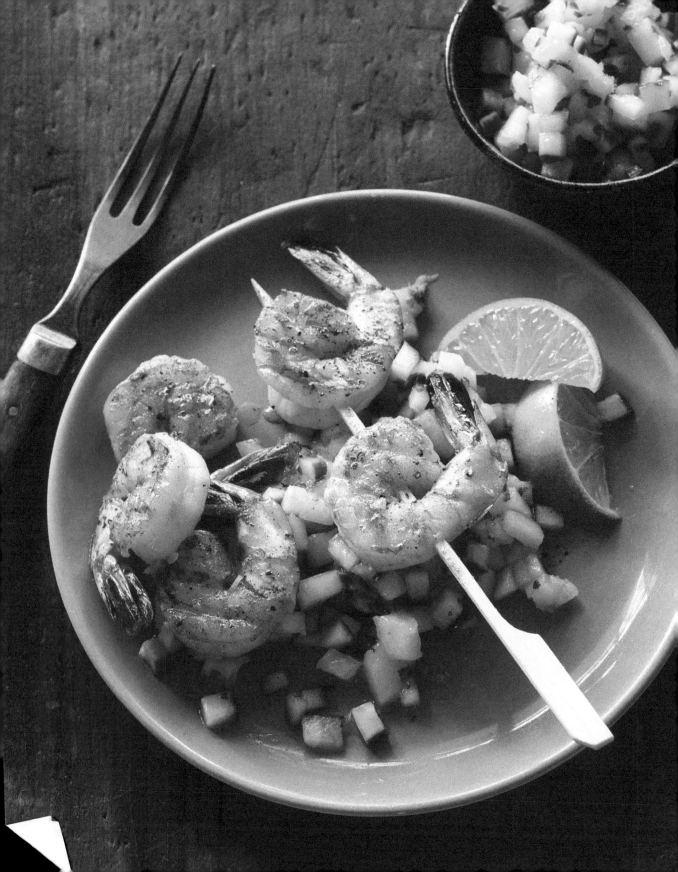

CHAPTER SEVEN

Fish and Shellfish

Opposite: Grilled Shrimp with Mango-Cucumber Salsa, page 119

In this luscious dish, flaky white fish floats in a golden broth of turmeric and ginger. The bits of potato give the soup body, but if you're sensitive to nightshades or following a paleo diet, simply replace the potatoes with cauliflower florets.

ELEGANT WHITE FISH SOUP

SERVES 4 / PREP TIME: 10 MINUTES / COOK TIME: 15 MINUTES

SOY-FREE

GLUTEN-FREE

NUT-FREE

MEDITERRANEAN

1 tablespoon extra-virgin olive oil

1 leek, sliced

1 teaspoon ground turmeric

1 teaspoon minced fresh ginger root

4 small new potatoes, scrubbed and quartered

4 cups vegetable broth

1½ pounds white fish fillets (cod, haddock, or pollock are all good choices), cut into 1-inch pieces

1 teaspoon salt

¼ teaspoon freshly ground black pepper

1 tablespoon chopped fresh parsley

1. In a Dutch oven, heat the oil over high heat.
2. Add the leek and sauté for 3 minutes. Add the turmeric, ginger root, and potatoes and sauté for 1 minute.
3. In the Dutch oven, bring the broth to a boil. Reduce to a simmer and simmer until the potatoes are tender, about 5 minutes.
4. Add the fish and cook for an additional 5 minutes. Add the salt, pepper, and parsley and serve.

RECIPE TIP: Benjamin Franklin once wrote, "Fish and visitors smell after three days." In line with that witticism, and because this soup does not keep well, you should eat this soup within 3 days of making it.

INGREDIENT TIP: If you like shellfish, both shrimp and scallops would work well in this dish.

NUTRITIONAL INFORMATION PER SERVING: Calories: 220; Total Fat: 5g; Total Carbohydrates: 11g; Sugar: 1g; Fiber: 2g; Protein: 31g; Sodium: 830mg

Mushrooms are getting a lot of attention in the medical community for their immune-boosting properties. Shiitake mushrooms are the stars of the grocery store mushrooms for healing purposes, but they can be expensive, so feel free to substitute regular button or cremini mushrooms, which are also very beneficial.

WHITE FISH WITH MUSHROOMS

SERVES 4 / PREP TIME: 15 MINUTES / COOK TIME: 18 MINUTES

SOY-FREE

GLUTEN-FREE

NUT-FREE

PALEO

MEDITERRANEAN

1 leek, thinly sliced

1 teaspoon minced fresh ginger root

1 garlic clove, minced

½ cup sliced shiitake mushrooms

½ cup dry white wine

1 tablespoon toasted sesame oil

4 (6-ounce) white fish fillets (such as cod, haddock, or pollock)

1 teaspoon salt

⅛ teaspoon freshly ground black pepper

1. Preheat the oven to 375°F.
2. Combine the leek, ginger root, garlic, mushrooms, wine, and sesame oil in a 9-by-13-inch baking pan. Toss well to combine.
3. Bake for 10 minutes.
4. Set the fish on top of the mushrooms. Add the salt and pepper, cover with aluminum foil, and bake until the fish is firm, 5 to 8 minutes. Serve.

RECIPE TIP: Salmon and swordfish also work well in this recipe. As with most cooked fish, eat within 3 days of making.

NUTRITIONAL INFORMATION PER SERVING (using cod): Calories: 210; Total Fat: 5g; Total Carbohydrates: 5g; Sugar: 1g; Fiber: 1g; Protein: 31g; Sodium: 680mg

Trout is typically available year-round. Since it's a freshwater fish, it tends to be enjoyable even to people who claim they don't like fish. The trout is baked on a bed of spinach, so all you need is a side dish to round out dinner, like Rosemary Wild Rice (page 58).

SPICED TROUT AND SPINACH

SERVES 4 / PREP TIME: 10 MINUTES / COOK TIME: 15 MINUTES

SOY-FREE

GLUTEN-FREE

NUT-FREE

PALEO

MEDITERRANEAN

Extra-virgin olive oil, for brushing

½ red onion, thinly sliced

1 (10-ounce) package frozen spinach, thawed

4 boneless trout fillets

1 teaspoon salt

¼ teaspoon chipotle powder

¼ teaspoon garlic powder

2 tablespoons fresh lemon juice

1. Preheat the oven to 375°F. Brush a 9-by-13-inch baking pan with olive oil.
2. Scatter the red onion and spinach in the pan.
3. Lay the trout fillets over the spinach.
4. Sprinkle the salt, chipotle powder, and garlic powder over the fish.
5. Cover with aluminum foil and bake until the trout is firm, about 15 minutes.
6. Drizzle with the lemon juice and serve.

SUBSTITUTION TIP: Other mild white fish like cod, halibut, or pollock would also work well in this dish. Stronger-tasting fish will permeate the spinach, compromising its natural flavor.

RECIPE TIP: Enjoy within 3 days of making.

NUTRITIONAL INFORMATION PER SERVING: Calories: 160; Total Fat: 7g; Total Carbohydrates: 5g; Sugar: 1g; Fiber: 2g; Protein: 19g; Sodium: 670mg

This dish offers a great opportunity to use up leftover rice and vegetables. Carrots, celery, broccoli, peppers, cauliflower, you name it—throw it into this potpourri! If you're avoiding soy and nuts, omit the soy sauce and toasted almonds. If salt is a concern for you, omit the soy sauce to lower the recipe's sodium content.

SMOKED TROUT FRIED RICE

SERVES 4 / PREP TIME: 10 MINUTES / COOK TIME: 10 MINUTES

GLUTEN-FREE

MEDITERRANEAN

2 tablespoons toasted sesame oil

4 scallions, thinly sliced

1 teaspoon minced fresh ginger root

1 garlic clove, minced

1/8 teaspoon red pepper flakes

2 cups baby spinach

1/2 cup chicken or vegetable broth

4 cups cooked brown rice

1 teaspoon low-sodium soy sauce (optional)

8 ounces smoked trout, flaked

1/4 cup toasted slivered almonds (optional)

1. Heat the sesame oil in a large skillet over high heat.
2. Add the scallions, ginger root, garlic, red pepper flakes, spinach, and broth. Sauté until the spinach has wilted, about 2 minutes.
3. Add the rice and stir to combine. Stir in the soy sauce (if using) and the trout.
4. Garnish with the almonds, (if using) and serve.

SUBSTITUTION TIP: This recipe can be made with leftover white rice instead of brown. Store in the refrigerator for up to 5 days.

NUTRITIONAL INFORMATION PER SERVING (including soy sauce and almonds): Calories: 430; Total Fat: 15g; Total Carbohydrates: 49g; Sugar: 2g; Fiber: 5g; Protein: 26g; Sodium: 2670mg

Oven-poached salmon is the star of this light salad. Perfect for spring when crisp, colorful radishes are in season, this delightful dish is best served cold. If you don't have escarole (also known as curly endive), you can substitute arugula, chopped radicchio, or baby spinach. If salt is a health concern for you, omit the salt from step two to lower the recipe's sodium content.

DILL SALMON WITH CUCUMBER-RADISH SALAD

SERVES 4 / PREP TIME: 10 MINUTES / COOK TIME: 20 MINUTES

SOY-FREE

GLUTEN-FREE

NUT-FREE

PALEO

MEDITERRANEAN

1 tablespoon extra-virgin olive oil, plus more for brushing

4 (3- to 4-ounce) boneless salmon fillets

2 or 3 dill sprigs, plus 2 teaspoons minced dill fronds

1 shallot, sliced

½ cup dry white wine

2 teaspoons salt, divided

¼ teaspoon freshly ground black pepper

2 cups sliced escarole

8 radishes, quartered

1 English cucumber, seeded and chopped

1 tablespoon fresh lemon juice, plus extra sliced lemons for garnish

1. Preheat the oven to 375°F. Brush a 9-inch square baking pan with olive oil.
2. Place the salmon fillets, skin-side down, in the pan. Scatter the dill sprigs and shallot over the fish, then add the wine, 1 teaspoon of salt, and the pepper.
3. Cover with aluminum foil and bake until the fish is firm, 20 to 25 minutes.
4. Transfer the salmon fillets to a plate and let them cool completely. Discard the remaining contents of the pan.

5. In a medium bowl, combine the escarole, radishes, cucumber, and minced dill. Add the lemon juice, 1 tablespoon of olive oil, and the remaining 1 teaspoon of salt. Toss well.

6. Mound the salad on four plates, top with the salmon, and garnish with the lemon slices. Serve.

SUBSTITUTION TIP: This oven-poaching technique works equally well with boneless, skinless chicken breast. If cooking chicken this way, increase the cooking time to 35 minutes.

NUTRITIONAL INFORMATION PER SERVING: Calories: 361; Total Fat: 22.9g; Total Carbohydrates: 5.4g; Sugar: 2g; Fiber: 0.7g; Protein: 27.5g; Sodium: 3,177mg

Miso is a fermented soybean paste with a salty, sweet, and savory flavor. The miso marinade used in this recipe also works well on vegetables—miso-marinated Brussels sprouts may become one of your favorite ways to eat this vegetable.

MISO BAKED SALMON

SERVES 4 / PREP TIME: 10 MINUTES / COOK TIME: 15 TO 20 MINUTES

GLUTEN-FREE

NUT-FREE

MEDITERRANEAN

¼ cup white miso

¼ cup apple cider

1 tablespoon unseasoned white rice vinegar

1 tablespoon toasted sesame oil

⅛ teaspoon ground ginger

4 (3- to 4-ounce) boneless salmon fillets

1 scallion, sliced

⅛ teaspoon red pepper flakes

1. Preheat the oven to 375°F.
2. In a small bowl whisk together the miso, cider, rice vinegar, sesame oil, and ginger. If the mixture is too thick, thin with a small amount of water.
3. Place the salmon fillets, skin-side down, in a 9-inch square baking pan. Pour the miso sauce over the salmon to coat evenly.
4. Bake until the salmon is firm, 15 to 20 minutes.
5. Top with the scallions and red pepper flakes and serve.

RECIPE TIP: The miso marinade can be made ahead and stored in the refrigerator for several weeks. Eat the salmon within 3 days of making.

NUTRITIONAL INFORMATION PER SERVING: Calories: 250; Total Fat: 15g; Total Carbohydrates: 8g; Sugar: 4g; Fiber: 1g; Protein: 21g; Sodium: 820mg

This recipe pulls together in a snap if you use already cooked salmon and quinoa. Substitute any seasonal vegetables you like. If you're not allergic to nuts, the almonds provide extra flavor and crunch.

QUINOA SALMON BOWL

SERVES 4 / PREP TIME: 15 MINUTES

SOY-FREE

GLUTEN-FREE

MEDITERRANEAN

4 cups cooked quinoa

1 pound cooked salmon, flaked

3 cups arugula

6 radishes, thinly sliced

1 zucchini, sliced into half moons

3 scallions, minced

½ cup almond oil

1 tablespoon apple cider vinegar

1 teaspoon Sriracha or other hot sauce (or more if you like it spicy)

1 teaspoon salt

½ cup toasted slivered almonds (optional)

1. Combine the quinoa, salmon, arugula, radishes, zucchini, and scallions in a large bowl.
2. Add the almond oil, vinegar, Sriracha, and salt and mix well.
3. Divide the mixture among four serving bowls, garnish with the toasted almonds (if using), and serve.

SUBSTITUTION TIP: To make this recipe vegan, simply omit the salmon.

INGREDIENT TIP: If you can't find cooked quinoa, it's a cinch to make. In a medium saucepan, combine 1 cup quinoa, 1 teaspoon salt, 1 teaspoon extra-virgin olive oil, and 2 cups water or broth. Bring to a boil, reduce to a simmer, and cook, partially covered, for 20 minutes. Fluff the quinoa and serve. If you find quinoa to be a little bitter, rinsing it in water before cooking will help.

NUTRITIONAL INFORMATION PER SERVING: Calories: 790; Total Fat: 52g; Total Carbohydrates: 45g; Sugar: 4g; Fiber: 8g; Protein: 37g; Sodium: 680mg

Coleslaw can be an overlooked high-nutrition meal option, but the prepared coleslaw sold in most grocery store deli sections is loaded with additives and stabilizers. Instead, grab a package of shredded cabbage, often labeled as coleslaw mix, and add cooked shrimp to make this tasty, healthy meal a breeze.

SHRIMP COLESLAW

SERVES 4 / PREP TIME: 10 MINUTES, PLUS 30 MINUTES TO CHILL

SOY-FREE

GLUTEN-FREE

NUT-FREE

PALEO

MEDITERRANEAN

1 pound frozen cooked shrimp, thawed

1 (8-ounce) package shredded cabbage

3 scallions, sliced

3 tangerines, peeled and sectioned

3 tablespoons toasted sesame oil

2 tablespoons unseasoned white rice vinegar

2 teaspoons grated fresh ginger root

⅛ teaspoon red pepper flakes

3 tablespoons chopped fresh cilantro

1 avocado, peeled, pitted, and sliced

¼ cup toasted slivered almonds (optional)

1. In a large bowl, combine the shrimp, cabbage, scallions, tangerines, sesame oil, vinegar, ginger root, and red pepper flakes. Mix well and chill for at least 30 minutes for the dressing to slightly wilt the cabbage.
2. Top with the cilantro, avocado, and almonds (if using) just before serving.

RECIPE TIP: Instead of purchasing pre-shredded cabbage, you can experiment with your own coleslaw veggie mix. Savoy cabbage, bok choy, and thinly sliced Brussels sprouts are all super, crunchy vegetables to make slaw with. Without adding the cilantro, avocado, and almonds, this salad will keep for up to 3 days in the refrigerator. Add the cilantro, avocado, and almonds just before serving.

NUTRITIONAL INFORMATION PER SERVING (including almonds): Calories: 380; Total Fat: 21g; Total Carbohydrates: 19g; Sugar: 10g; Fiber: 6g; Protein: 29g; Sodium: 1,090mg

Get the largest shrimp you can find—they're easier to skewer. Let the shrimp sit in the marinade for at least 15 minutes prior to cooking. If salt is a health concern for you, omit the salt from the marinade to lower the recipe's sodium content.

GRILLED SHRIMP WITH MANGO-CUCUMBER SALSA

SERVES 4 / PREP TIME: 15 MINUTES, PLUS 15 MINUTES TO MARINATE / COOK TIME: 10 MINUTES

SOY-FREE

GLUTEN-FREE

NUT-FREE

PALEO

MEDITERRANEAN

For the shrimp

¼ cup extra-virgin olive oil

3 tablespoons fresh lime juice, plus extra lime wedges for garnish

1 teaspoon salt

⅛ teaspoon chipotle powder

1½ pounds uncooked shrimp, peeled and deveined

For the salsa

1 large mango, peeled, pitted, and cubed

1 small cucumber, diced

1 scallion, sliced

1 tablespoon fresh lime juice

1 tablespoon extra-virgin olive oil

¼ teaspoon salt

1. In a shallow baking dish, combine the olive oil, lime juice, salt, and chipotle powder. Add the shrimp, toss to combine, and let marinate for at least 15 minutes at room temperature or up to 2 hours in the refrigerator.
2. Meanwhile, in a small bowl, combine all the salsa ingredients. Store in the refrigerator until ready to serve.
3. When ready to cook, skewer the shrimp, fitting as many as you can on each skewer.
4. Heat a stove top grill or skillet over high heat. When the grill is hot, lay the skewers on the grill, being careful not to crowd them. Cook until the shrimp are pale pink and firm to the touch, 2 to 3 minutes.
5. Serve the shrimp skewers over a bed of salsa, with lime wedges for squeezing.

RECIPE TIP: Soaking wooden skewers in water will make them less likely to burn on the grill.

NUTRITIONAL INFORMATION PER SERVING: Calories: 340; Total Fat: 19g; Total Carbohydrates: 18g; Sugar: 13g; Fiber: 2g; Protein: 24g; Sodium: 1,690mg

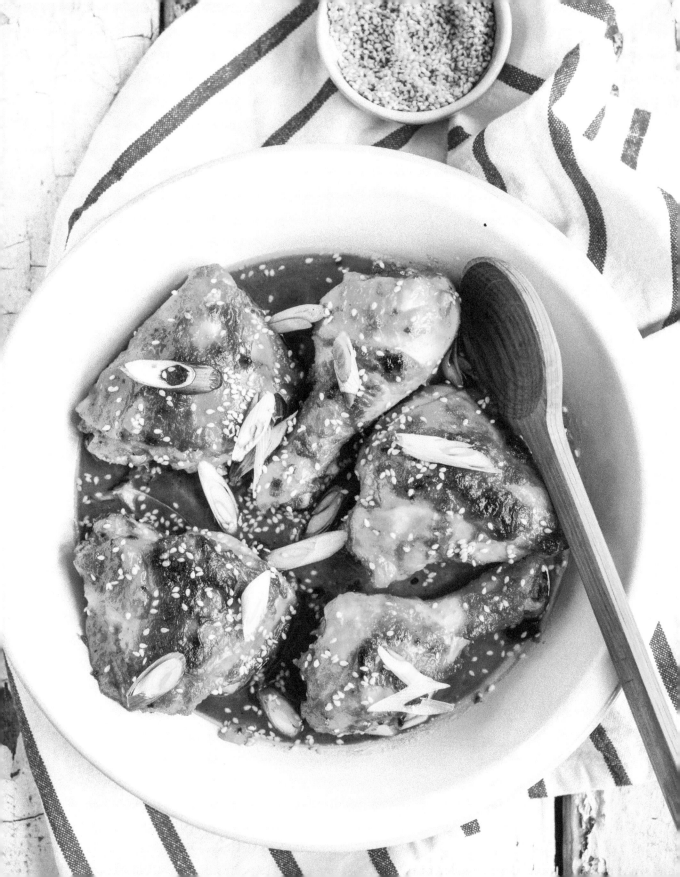

CHAPTER EIGHT

Poultry and Meat

Opposite: Sesame Miso Chicken, page 123

Two anti-inflammatory darlings, turmeric and coriander, flavor this comforting slow cooker dish, with ginger adding a little extra something special. Chicken broth and coconut milk blend nicely into a creamy sauce. Serve with Roasted–Butternut Squash Mash (page 57) or steamed brown rice.

COMFORTING CHICKEN STEW

SERVES 4 TO 6 / PREP TIME: 15 MINUTES / COOK TIME: 4 HOURS

SOY-FREE

GLUTEN-FREE

NUT-FREE

PALEO

MEDITERRANEAN

1 tablespoon extra-virgin olive oil

3 pounds boneless, skinless chicken thighs

1 large onion, thinly sliced

2 garlic cloves, thinly sliced

1 teaspoon minced fresh ginger root

2 teaspoons ground turmeric

1 teaspoon whole coriander seeds, lightly crushed

1 teaspoon salt

¼ teaspoon freshly ground black pepper

2 cups chicken broth

1 cup unsweetened coconut milk

¼ cup chopped fresh cilantro (optional)

1. Drizzle the oil into a slow cooker.
2. Add the chicken, onion, garlic, ginger root, turmeric, coriander, salt, pepper, chicken broth, and coconut milk, and toss to combine.
3. Cover and cook on high for 4 hours. Garnish with the chopped cilantro (if using) and serve.

INGREDIENT TIP: If your market sells fresh turmeric root, it's worth getting, since the healing properties of turmeric are stronger in the root than in ground turmeric. Simply substitute 2 teaspoons grated fresh turmeric root for every 1 teaspoon ground turmeric.

NUTRITIONAL INFORMATION PER SERVING (6 portions): Calories: 370; Total Fat: 19g; Total Carbohydrates: 4g; Sugar: 1g; Fiber: 1g; Protein: 46g; Sodium: 770mg

Bone-in chicken thighs are inexpensive and ideal for the slow cooker, because it's almost impossible to overcook them. From the long, slow cook emerges a rich delicious sauce, with the miso providing a salty sweetness. Serve over a bed of brown rice and sautéed bok choy.

SESAME MISO CHICKEN

SERVES 4 TO 6 / PREP TIME: 10 MINUTES / COOK TIME: 4 HOURS

GLUTEN-FREE

NUT-FREE

MEDITERRANEAN

¼ cup white miso

2 tablespoons coconut oil, melted

2 tablespoons honey

1 tablespoon unseasoned rice wine vinegar

2 garlic cloves, thinly sliced

1 teaspoon minced fresh ginger root

1 cup chicken broth

8 boneless, skinless chicken thighs

2 scallions, sliced

1 tablespoon sesame seeds

1. In a slow cooker, combine the miso, coconut oil, honey, rice wine vinegar, garlic, and ginger root, mixing well.
2. Add the chicken and toss to combine. Cover and cook on high for 4 hours.
3. Transfer the chicken and sauce to a serving dish. Garnish with the scallions and sesame seeds and serve.

RECIPE TIP: You can use chicken drumsticks instead of thighs—an equally tasty and economical alternative. Store leftovers in the refrigerator for up to a week.

NUTRITIONAL INFORMATION PER SERVING (4 portions): Calories: 320; Total Fat: 15g; Total Carbohydrates: 17g; Sugar: 11g; Fiber: 1g; Protein: 32g; Sodium: 1,020mg

Our favorite way to eat these savory burgers is on a bed of lettuce with ripe tomatoes, thinly sliced red onions, and pitted olives. But you can also enjoy them the traditional way, inside a bun with lettuce, tomato, and a juicy, anti-inflammatory pickle.

GINGER TURKEY BURGERS

SERVES 4 / PREP TIME: 10 MINUTES / COOK TIME: 10 MINUTES

SOY-FREE

GLUTEN-FREE

NUT-FREE

PALEO

MEDITERRANEAN

1½ pounds ground turkey

1 large egg, lightly beaten

2 tablespoons coconut or almond flour

½ cup finely chopped onion

1 garlic clove, minced

2 teaspoons minced fresh ginger root

1 tablespoon fresh cilantro

1 teaspoon salt

¼ teaspoon freshly ground black pepper

1 tablespoon extra-virgin olive oil

1. In a medium bowl, combine the ground turkey, egg, flour, onion, garlic, ginger root, cilantro, salt, and pepper and mix well.
2. Form the turkey mixture into four patties.
3. Heat the olive oil in a large skillet over medium-high heat.
4. Cook the burgers, flipping once, until firm to the touch, 3 to 4 minutes on each side. Serve.

RECIPE TIP: Store leftovers in the fridge for a week or freeze for longer.

SUBSTITUTION TIP: The flour used in this recipe helps the burgers keep their shape; if you're not sensitive to gluten, you can use bread crumbs instead.

NUTRITIONAL INFORMATION PER SERVING: Calories: 320; Total Fat: 20g; Total Carbohydrates: 2g; Sugar: 1g; Fiber: <1g; Protein: 34g; Sodium: 720mg

This dish is a soothing mixture of turkey and mushrooms cooked in broth and wine. If you're not otherwise diet-restricted, try serving it over cooked wide noodles topped with a generous shaving of Parmesan cheese.

MUSHROOM TURKEY THIGHS

SERVES 4 / PREP TIME: 15 MINUTES / COOK TIME: 4 HOURS

SOY-FREE

GLUTEN-FREE

NUT-FREE

PALEO

MEDITERRANEAN

1 tablespoon extra-virgin olive oil

2 turkey thighs

2 cups button or cremini mushrooms, sliced

1 large onion, sliced

1 garlic clove, sliced

1 rosemary sprig

1 teaspoon salt

¼ teaspoon freshly ground black pepper

2 cups chicken broth

½ cup dry red wine

1. Drizzle the olive oil into a slow cooker. Add the turkey thighs, mushrooms, onion, garlic, rosemary sprig, salt, and pepper. Pour in the chicken broth and wine. Cover and cook on high for 4 hours.
2. Remove and discard the rosemary sprig. Use a slotted spoon to transfer the thighs to a plate and allow them to cool for several minutes for easier handling.
3. Cut the meat from the bones, stir the meat into the mushrooms, and serve.

RECIPE TIP: If you have time, you can add even more flavor by browning the turkey thighs in a little bit of oil in a skillet before adding them to the slow cooker. Store leftovers in the refrigerator for up to a week or in the freezer for longer.

NUTRITIONAL INFORMATION PER SERVING: Calories: 280; Total Fat: 9g; Total Carbohydrates: 3g; Sugar: 1g; Fiber: <1g; Protein: 43g; Sodium: 850mg

Chocolate in chili? Yep—unsweetened cocoa contains flavonoids that can help improve blood flow. Just a touch adds nice depth to sauces and seasonings, like spice rubs for beef and pork. This chili fits the paleo diet since it doesn't contain beans, but if you want to, by all means add a 15-ounce can of black beans, drained and rinsed, at the very end of the cooking time.

CHOCOLATE CHILI

SERVES 4 TO 6 / PREP TIME: 15 MINUTES / COOK TIME: 45 MINUTES

SOY-FREE

GLUTEN-FREE

NUT-FREE

PALEO

MEDITERRANEAN

1 tablespoon extra-virgin olive oil

1 pound lean ground beef

1 large onion, chopped

2 garlic cloves, minced

1 tablespoon unsweetened cocoa

1½ teaspoons chili powder

1 teaspoon salt

½ teaspoon ground cumin

2 cups chicken broth

1 cup tomato sauce

1. In a Dutch oven, heat the oil over high heat. Add the ground beef and brown well, about 5 minutes.
2. Add the onion, garlic, cocoa, chili powder, salt, and cumin and cook, stirring, for an additional minute.
3. Add the chicken broth and tomato sauce and bring to a boil. Reduce the heat to a simmer, cover, and cook, stirring occasionally, for 30 to 40 minutes. If the sauce becomes too thick as it cooks, add more chicken broth or water to thin it.
4. Ladle into bowls and serve.

RECIPE TIP: This dish can be stored for up to a week in the refrigerator or in the freezer for even longer.

SUBSTITUTION TIP: If you are reactive to nightshades, omit the tomato sauce and use a total of 3 cups chicken broth.

NUTRITIONAL INFORMATION PER SERVING (4 portions): Calories: 370; Total Fat: 27g; Total Carbohydrates: 9g; Sugar: 4g; Fiber: 2g; Protein: 23g; Sodium: 1,010mg

If you haven't tried grass-fed beef, this is a good recipe to start with. Grass-fed beef has great flavor, but the meat can be a little tough. Marinating it before cooking helps tenderize it. This recipe calls for pan-searing, but an outdoor grill works just as well.

GARLIC-MUSTARD STEAK

SERVES 4 / PREP TIME: 10 MINUTES, PLUS 30 MINUTES TO MARINATE / COOK TIME: 10 MINUTES

SOY-FREE

GLUTEN-FREE

NUT-FREE

PALEO

MEDITERRANEAN

½ cup extra-virgin olive oil

½ cup balsamic vinegar

2 tablespoons Dijon mustard

2 garlic cloves, minced

1 teaspoon chopped fresh rosemary

1 teaspoon salt

¼ teaspoon freshly ground black pepper

4 (6-ounce) boneless grass-fed steaks, about ½ inch thick

1. In a shallow baking dish, whisk together the olive oil, balsamic vinegar, Dijon, garlic, rosemary, salt, and pepper.
2. Add the steaks and turn them to coat well with the marinade. Cover and let the steaks marinate for 30 minutes at room temperature or up to 2 hours in the refrigerator.
3. Heat a large skillet over high heat.
4. Remove the steaks from the marinade and blot them with a paper towel to remove any excess marinade.
5. Cook the steaks, flipping once, until nicely browned, 2 to 3 minutes on each side.
6. Let the steaks rest for 5 minutes before serving.

RECIPE TIP: The marinade can be made up to a week ahead and can also be used on lamb chops or chicken. Store leftover steak in the refrigerator for up to a week.

NUTRITIONAL INFORMATION PER SERVING: Calories: 480; Total Fat: 31g; Total Carbohydrates: 3g; Sugar: 2g; Fiber: 0g; Protein: 48g; Sodium: 390mg

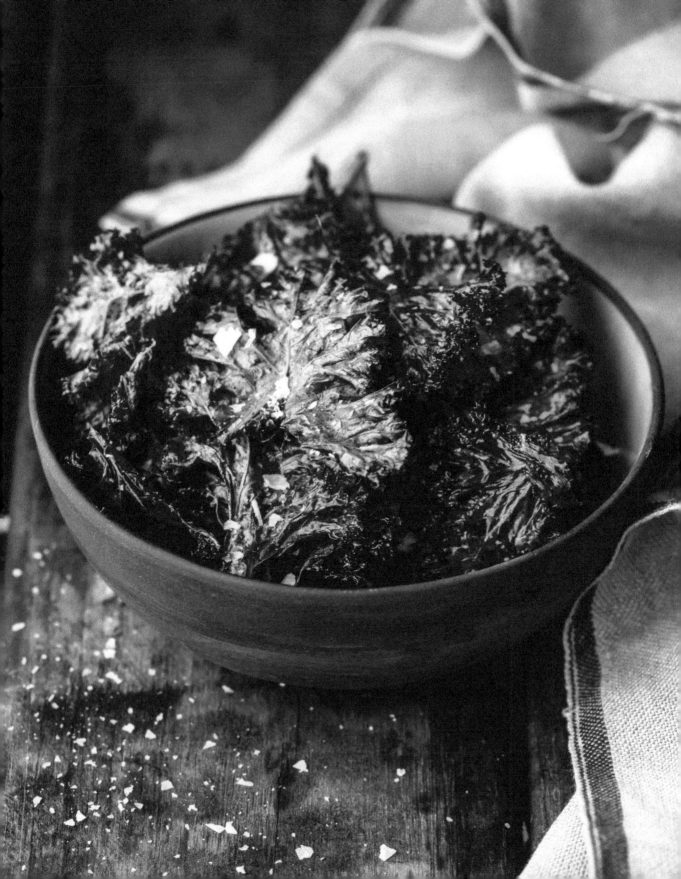

CHAPTER NINE

Snacks and Sweets

Opposite: Kale Chips, page 130

Even though kale chips are readily available at the grocery store, they can be expensive. This recipe makes delicious chips at a fraction of the price. Better yet, when you make your own, you know exactly what's in them and are assured you're getting maximum nutrition. If you like it spicy, add a pinch of red pepper flakes to the kale before baking.

KALE CHIPS

SERVES 4 / PREP TIME: 15 MINUTES / COOK TIME: 20 MINUTES

SOY-FREE

GLUTEN-FREE

NUT-FREE

VEGAN

PALEO

MEDITERRANEAN

1 large bunch kale, washed and thoroughly dried, stems removed, leaves cut into 2-inch pieces

2 tablespoons extra-virgin olive oil

1 teaspoon sea salt

1. Preheat the oven to 275°F.
2. In a large bowl, use your hands to mix the kale and olive oil until the kale is evenly coated.
3. Transfer the kale to a large baking sheet and sprinkle the sea salt over it.
4. Bake, turning the kale leaves once halfway through, until crispy, about 20 minutes.

RECIPE TIP: It's best to enjoy these kale chips within 24 hours of making them, because they lose their crunch quickly. Keep them in an airtight container at room temperature.

NUTRITIONAL INFORMATION PER SERVING: Calories: 88; Total Fat: 7.2g; Total Carbohydrates: 5.7g; Sugar: 1.3g; Fiber: 2g; Protein: 1.9g; Sodium: 605mg

This hummus-esque recipe is the base for the Whole-Grain Toast with Chickpea Paste, Avocado, and Grilled Tomato (page 95). Fast and easy, enjoy this super-nutritious high-protein spread on toast, or as a yummy dip for fresh vegetable sticks.

CHICKPEA PASTE

MAKES ABOUT 2 CUPS / PREP TIME: 15 MINUTES, PLUS 30 MINUTES TO SIT

SOY-FREE

GLUTEN-FREE

NUT-FREE

VEGAN

MEDITERRANEAN

1 (15-ounce) can chickpeas, drained and rinsed

¼ cup extra-virgin olive oil

¼ cup fresh lemon juice

¼ cup minced onion

1 garlic clove, minced

1 teaspoon sea salt

½ teaspoon ground cumin

¼ teaspoon red pepper flakes

1. In a medium bowl, use a potato masher to mash the chickpeas until they are mostly broken up.
2. Add the olive oil, lemon juice, onion, garlic, salt, cumin, and red pepper flakes and continue mashing until you have a slightly chunky paste. Let sit for 30 minutes at room temperature for the flavors to develop, then serve.

RECIPE TIP: This recipe can also be made with black or white beans. Store in the refrigerator for about a week.

NUTRITIONAL INFORMATION PER SERVING (¼ cup): Calories: 110; Total Fat: 8g; Total Carbohydrates: 10g; Sugar: 2g; Fiber: 2g; Protein: 3g; Sodium: 290mg

Raw, unsalted nuts are the best nuts to eat—even when toasted—
because they are closest to their whole state. Nuts are loaded with
protein and a great source of fiber, vitamins, and minerals.

SPICED NUTS

MAKES ABOUT 2 CUPS / PREP TIME: 10 MINUTES / COOK TIME: 15 MINUTES

SOY-FREE

GLUTEN-FREE

VEGAN

PALEO

MEDITERRANEAN

1 cup almonds

½ cup walnuts

¼ cup sunflower seeds

¼ cup pumpkin seeds

1 teaspoon ground turmeric

½ teaspoon ground cumin

¼ teaspoon garlic powder

¼ teaspoon red pepper flakes

1. Preheat the oven to 350°F.
2. Combine all the ingredients in a medium bowl and mix well.
3. Spread the nuts evenly on a rimmed baking sheet and bake until lightly toasted, 10 to 15 minutes.
4. Cool completely before serving or storing.

RECIPE TIP: You can make this recipe with any assortment of nuts or spices you wish—test out your many options! Store at room temperature for up to 10 days.

NUTRITIONAL INFORMATION PER SERVING (¼ cup): Calories: 180; Total Fat: 16g; Total Carbohydrates: 7g; Sugar: 1g; Fiber: 3g; Protein: 6g; Sodium: <5mg

Lassi, a delicious drink made with yogurt, can be sweet or not. The sweet version of lassi, which we're presenting here, is usually made with mangos. This recipe calls for a combination of yogurt and coconut milk—the yogurt provides the traditional tartness and coconut milk adds sweetness.

COCONUT-MANGO LASSI

SERVES 2 / PREP TIME: 10 MINUTES

SOY-FREE

GLUTEN-FREE

VEGETARIAN

PALEO

MEDITERRANEAN

1½ cups frozen mango chunks

1 cup unsweetened coconut milk

1 cup ice cubes

½ cup plain yogurt

1 tablespoon honey

Pinch ground cardamom

1. Combine the mango, coconut milk, ice cubes, yogurt, and honey in a blender and blend until smooth.
2. Pour into two tall glasses. Sprinkle a little ground cardamom over each drink and serve.

SUBSTITUTION TIP: If you're vegan, try substituting coconut yogurt for the plain yogurt and maple syrup for the honey.

NUTRITIONAL INFORMATION PER SERVING: Calories: 370; Total Fat: 26g; Total Carbohydrates: 32g; Sugar: 27g; Fiber: 2g; Protein: 8g; Sodium: 30mg

We first discovered avocado fudge at a store that was, interestingly, completely devoted to it. The store had at least ten different flavors of avocado fudge, and not all of them even contained chocolate. Their recipe was a true candy recipe, a complex process involving cooking sugar and water to the "soft ball" stage and adding ingredients for flavor and texture. This is a much more simplified version!

AVOCADO FUDGE

16 PIECES / PREP TIME: 15 MINUTES, PLUS 3 HOURS TO CHILL

SOY-FREE

GLUTEN-FREE

NUT-FREE

VEGAN

MEDITERRANEAN

1½ cup bittersweet chocolate chips

¼ cup coconut oil

1 ripe avocado, peeled and pitted

½ teaspoon sea salt

1. Line an 8-inch square baking pan with waxed or parchment paper.
2. In a double boiler (not the microwave), melt the chocolate and coconut oil.
3. Once melted, transfer to the bowl of a food processor and let them cool a bit. (If the chocolate is too hot when combined with the avocado, the mixture will separate.) Add the avocado and process until smooth.
4. Spoon the mixture into the lined pan, sprinkle with the sea salt, and chill for 3 hours. Cut into 16 pieces and serve.

RECIPE TIP: The chocolate in this recipe needs to melt slowly and gently. If you don't have a double boiler, you can make one. Just pour about 1½ inches of water into a medium pot, bring to a boil, and turn the heat off. Put the chocolate and coconut oil in a small heat-resistant bowl and set it in the pot of hot water, stirring occasionally to melt the chocolate. Store leftover avocado fudge in the refrigerator or freezer.

NUTRITIONAL INFORMATION PER SERVING (1 piece): Calories: 120; Total Fat: 9g; Total Carbohydrates: 11g; Sugar: 9g; Fiber: 2g; Protein: 1g; Sodium: 80mg

Slightly sweet, with a touch of cinnamon, these pears are delicious served over yogurt and topped with the crunch of nuts. Try nuts instead of syrup with pancakes or waffles.

CARAMELIZED PEARS WITH YOGURT

SERVES 4 / PREP TIME: 15 MINUTES / COOK TIME: 10 MINUTES

SOY-FREE

GLUTEN-FREE

VEGETARIAN

PALEO

MEDITERRANEAN

1 tablespoon coconut oil

4 pears, peeled, cored, and quartered

2 tablespoons honey

1 teaspoon ground cinnamon

⅛ teaspoon sea salt

2 cups plain yogurt

¼ cup chopped toasted pecans (optional)

1. Heat the oil in a large skillet over medium-high heat.
2. Add the pears, honey, cinnamon, and salt, cover, and cook, stirring occasionally, until the fruit is tender, 4 to 5 minutes.
3. Uncover and let the sauce simmer for several more minutes to thicken.
4. Spoon the yogurt into four dessert bowls. Top with the warm pears, garnish with the pecans (if using), and serve.

RECIPE TIP: The pears can be made several days ahead and stored in the refrigerator until ready to serve. Reheat or simply enjoy cold.

SUBSTITUTION TIP: To make this dish vegan, use maple syrup instead of honey, and use a nondairy yogurt.

NUTRITIONAL INFORMATION PER SERVING (including pecans): Calories: 290; Total Fat: 11g; Total Carbohydrates: 41g; Sugar: 30g; Fiber: 6g; Protein: 12g; Sodium: 110mg

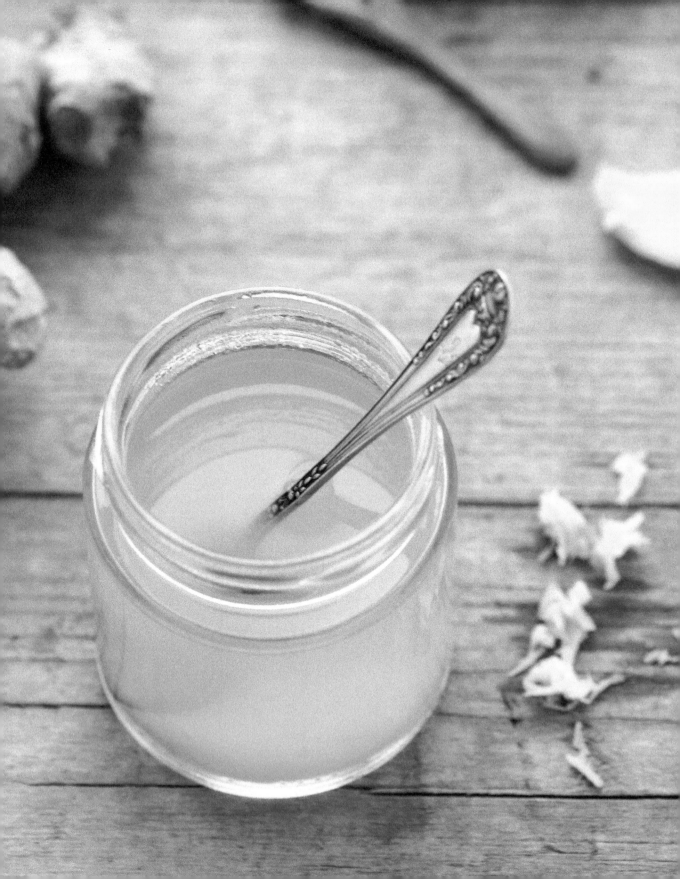

CHAPTER TEN

Sauces, Condiments, and Dressings

Opposite: Lemon-Ginger Honey, page 143

This is a high-protein spin on pesto, which can be used to give pasta and bean dishes a flavorful nutritional boost. When you're buying tofu, look for organic tofu, since soybean crops are often loaded with pesticides.

TOFU-BASIL SAUCE

MAKES ABOUT 2 CUPS / PREP TIME: 10 MINUTES

GLUTEN-FREE

VEGAN

MEDITERRANEAN

1 (12-ounce) package silken tofu

½ cup chopped fresh basil

2 garlic cloves, lightly crushed

½ cup almond butter

1 tablespoon fresh lemon juice

1 teaspoon salt

¼ teaspoon freshly ground black pepper

1. In a blender or food processor, combine the tofu, basil, garlic, almond butter, lemon juice, salt, and pepper. Process until smooth. If too thick, thin with a bit of water.
2. Refrigerate in an airtight container for up to 5 days.

SUBSTITUTION TIP: If you're sensitive to nuts, you can substitute tahini or sunflower seed butter for the almond butter.

NUTRITIONAL INFORMATION PER SERVING (8 portions): Calories: 120; Total Fat: 10g; Total Carbohydrates: 5g; Sugar: 1g; Fiber: 2g; Protein: 6g; Sodium: 290mg

Chutneys make a great addition to curries and soups, a condiment for grilled meats or fish, and a tasty topping for cooked grains. You can make chutneys out of nearly any fruits or vegetables. We chose apples for this flavorful recipe, because they have the perfect texture for chutney, and the pectin in apples is a digestive aid.

APPLE CHUTNEY

MAKES ABOUT 2 CUPS / PREP TIME: 10 MINUTES / COOK TIME: 10 MINUTES

SOY-FREE

GLUTEN-FREE

VEGETARIAN

PALEO

MEDITERRANEAN

1 tablespoon almond oil

4 apples, peeled, cored, and diced

1 small onion, diced

½ cup white raisins (optional)

1 tablespoon apple cider vinegar

1 tablespoon honey

1 teaspoon ground cinnamon

½ teaspoon ground cardamom

½ teaspoon ground ginger

½ teaspoon salt

1. In a medium saucepan, heat the oil over low heat.
2. Add the apples, onion, raisins (if using), vinegar, honey, cinnamon, cardamom, ginger, and salt. Cook briefly, just until the apples begin to release their juices. Bring to a simmer, cover, and cook until the apples are tender, 5 to 10 minutes.
3. Allow to cool completely before serving.

RECIPE TIP: This chutney can be stored in the refrigerator for several weeks. If you're vegan, substitute maple syrup for the honey.

INGREDIENT TIP: You can use any type of apples for this, but try to pair a low-sugar apple like Granny Smith with a sweeter, juicier apple like Braeburn for a more complex flavor.

NUTRITIONAL INFORMATION PER SERVING (¼ cup including raisins): Calories: 120; Total Fat: 2g; Total Carbohydrates: 24g; Sugar: 18; Fiber: 3g; Protein: 1g; Sodium: 150mg

It's culinary insurance having a spice mix on hand—and this one's anti-inflammatory. What could be more reassuring than knowing you need only turn to your pantry for an easy, customized solution to perk up a bland dish? In addition to using it to season meats, try sprinkling it over sweet potatoes or on top of avocado.

ZESTY SPICE RUB

MAKES ABOUT ½ CUP / PREP TIME: 10 MINUTES

SOY-FREE

GLUTEN-FREE

NUT-FREE

VEGAN

PALEO

MEDITERRANEAN

1 tablespoon ground turmeric

1 tablespoon ground ginger

1 tablespoon ground fennel seed

1 tablespoon coconut sugar (optional)

2 teaspoons salt

2 teaspoons onion powder

1 teaspoon garlic powder

1 teaspoon paprika

½ teaspoon freshly ground black pepper

1. Combine all the ingredients in a small bowl and mix well.
2. Store in an airtight container for up to 12 months.

RECIPE TIP: Add the coconut sugar only if you want your spice rub to have a hint of sweetness.

NUTRITIONAL INFORMATION PER SERVING (2 tablespoons): Calories: 20; Total Fat: 0g; Total Carbohydrates: 5g; Sugar: 0g; Fiber: 2g; Protein: 1g; Sodium: 1,160mg

You can call this the super-duper anti-inflammatory dressing, since it's loaded with some of nature's most potent anti-inflammatory elements: ginger, garlic, turmeric, and coriander. This dressing is called for in several recipes in this book, so consider making extra to keep on hand if you'll use it again within the week.

GINGER-TURMERIC DRESSING

MAKES ABOUT 1½ CUPS / PREP TIME: 10 MINUTES

SOY-FREE

GLUTEN-FREE

NUT-FREE

VEGAN

PALEO

MEDITERRANEAN

1 cup extra-virgin olive oil

¼ cup apple cider vinegar

½ teaspoon Dijon mustard

1 garlic clove, sliced

½ teaspoon minced fresh ginger root

1 teaspoon salt

½ teaspoon ground turmeric

¼ teaspoon ground coriander

¼ teaspoon freshly ground black pepper

1. In a blender or food processor, combine all the ingredients and process until smooth.
2. Refrigerate in an airtight container for up to a week.

RECIPE TIP: If you'd like to change up the essence a bit, add fresh herbs to this dressing. Cilantro, chives, and tarragon are all delicious in this recipe.

NUTRITIONAL INFORMATION PER SERVING (2 tablespoons): Calories: 160; Total Fat: 18g; Total Carbohydrates: 0g; Sugar: 0g; Fiber: 0g; Protein: 0g; Sodium: 200mg

This recipe makes a naturally delicious salad dressing, but it's also tasty as a sauce over steamed asparagus or broccoli. Try it as a marinade for poultry, meat, or seafood—see where it takes you!

LEMONY MUSTARD DRESSING

MAKES ABOUT 1½ CUPS / PREP TIME: 10 MINUTES

SOY-FREE

GLUTEN-FREE

NUT-FREE

VEGETARIAN

PALEO

MEDITERRANEAN

1 cup extra-virgin olive oil

¼ cup fresh lemon juice

1 tablespoon honey

1 teaspoon Dijon mustard

1 shallot, sliced

1 teaspoon grated lemon zest

1 teaspoon salt

¼ teaspoon pepper

1. In a blender or food processor, combine the olive oil, lemon juice, honey, Dijon, shallot, lemon zest, salt, and pepper. Process until smooth.
2. Refrigerate in an airtight container for up to 5 days.

SUBSTITUTION TIP: To make this recipe vegan, either omit the honey or substitute maple syrup.

NUTRITIONAL INFORMATION PER SERVING (2 tablespoons): Calories: 180; Total Fat: 20g; Total Carbohydrates: 2g; Sugar: 2g; Fiber: 0g; Protein: 0g; Sodium: 220mg

A "shrub" is the name for an old-fashioned mixture of sweet and sour to be added to cocktails or sparkling water for a refreshing drink. Our featured shrub is a mixture of lemon, ginger, and honey. In addition to its numerous applications in beverages, you can use it to marinate chicken or shrimp. If you love the taste of lemon, feel free to squeeze a bit more into this recipe.

LEMON-GINGER HONEY

MAKES ABOUT 1 CUP / PREP TIME: 10 MINUTES

SOY-FREE

GLUTEN-FREE

NUT-FREE

VEGETARIAN

PALEO

MEDITERRANEAN

1 cup water

¼ cup fresh lemon juice

2 tablespoons honey

2 teaspoons grated fresh ginger root

1. Combine all the ingredients in an airtight jar and shake until the honey is dissolved.
2. Refrigerate for 24 hours before using so the ginger can permeate the mixture.
3. Store in the refrigerator up to a week.

RECIPE TIP: To make a beverage, pour 2 tablespoons into a tall glass filled with ice. Add sparkling water or seltzer and serve.

NUTRITIONAL INFORMATION PER SERVING (2 tablespoons): Calories: 20; Total Fat: 0g; Total Carbohydrates: 5g; Sugar: 4g; Fiber: 0g; Protein: 0g; Sodium: 0mg

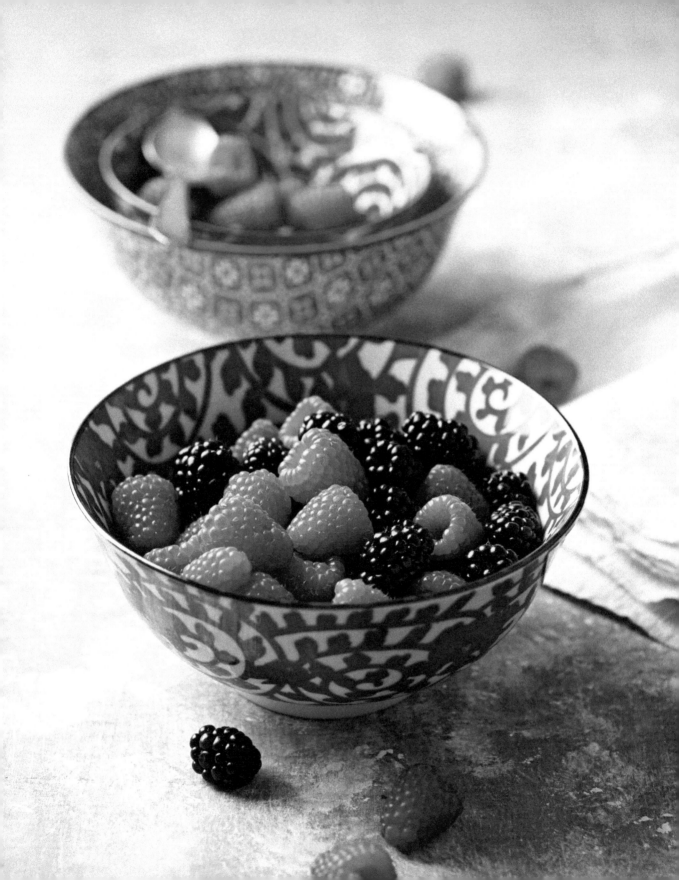

CONVERSION TABLES

Volume Equivalents (Liquid)

US Standard	US Standard (ounces)	Metric (approximate)
2 tablespoons	1 fl. oz.	30 mL
¼ cup	2 fl. oz.	60 mL
½ cup	4 fl. oz.	120 mL
1 cup	8 fl. oz.	240 mL
1½ cups	12 fl. oz.	355 mL
2 cups or 1 pint	16 fl. oz.	475 mL
4 cups or 1 quart	32 fl. oz.	1 L
1 gallon	128 fl. oz.	4 L

Oven Temperatures

Fahrenheit (F)	Celsius (C) (approximate)
250°F	120°C
300°F	150°C
325°F	165°C
350°F	180°C
375°F	190°C
400°F	200°C
425°F	220°C
450°F	230°C

Volume Equivalents (Dry)

US Standard	Metric (approximate)
⅛ teaspoon	0.5 mL
¼ teaspoon	1 mL
½ teaspoon	2 mL
¾ teaspoon	4 mL
1 teaspoon	5 mL
1 tablespoon	15 mL
¼ cup	59 mL
⅓ cup	79 mL
½ cup	118 mL
⅔ cup	156 mL
¾ cup	177 mL
1 cup	235 mL
2 cups or 1 pint	475 mL
3 cups	700 mL
4 cups or 1 quart	1 L

Weight Equivalents

US Standard	Metric (approximate)
½ ounce	15 g
1 ounce	30 g
2 ounces	60 g
4 ounces	115 g
8 ounces	225 g
12 ounces	340 g
16 ounces or 1 pound	455 g

THE DIRTY DOZEN AND THE CLEAN FIFTEEN

The Environmental Working Group (EWG) is a nonprofit, nonpartisan organization dedicated to protecting human health and the environment. Its mission is to empower people to live healthier lives in a healthier environment. This organization publishes an annual list of the twelve kinds of produce, in sequence, that have the highest amount of pesticide residue—the Dirty Dozen—as well as a list of the fifteen kinds of produce that have the least amount of pesticide residue—the Clean Fifteen.

THE DIRTY DOZEN

The 2016 Dirty Dozen includes the following produce. These are considered among the year's most important produce to buy organic:

Strawberries

Apples

Nectarines

Peaches

Celery

Grapes

Cherries

Spinach

Tomatoes

Bell peppers

Cherry tomatoes

Cucumbers

Kale/collard greens*

Hot peppers*

*The Dirty Dozen list contains two additional items— kale/collard greens and hot peppers—because they tend to contain trace levels of highly hazardous pesticides.

THE CLEAN FIFTEEN

The least critical to buy organically are the Clean Fifteen list. The following are on the 2016 list:

Avocados

Corn**

Pineapples

Cabbage

Sweet peas

Onions

Asparagus

Mangos

Papayas

Kiwi

Eggplant

Honeydew

Grapefruit

Cantaloupe

Cauliflower

** Some of the sweet corn sold in the United States are made from genetically engineered (GE) seedstock. Buy organic varieties of these crops to avoid GE produce.

RESOURCES

ARTHRITIS FOUNDATION
(arthritis.org)

THE CENTER FOR MINDFUL EATING
(thecenterformindfuleating.org)

JACK CHALLEM, THE
INFLAMMATION SYNDROME
(www.jackchallem.com/pages/inflammation
syndrome/inflammationsymdrome.html)

ENVIRONMENTAL WORKING GROUP
(ewg.org/consumer-guides)

LOSE IT!
(loseit.com)

OLDWAYS WHOLE GRAINS COUNCIL
(wholegrainscouncil.org)

THE PALEO DIET
(thepaleodiet.com)

REFERENCES

American Psychological Association. "Sleep and Stress." Accessed November 28, 2016. www.apa.org/news/press/releases/stress /2013/sleep.aspx.

Arthritis Foundation. "8 Food Ingredients that Can Cause Inflammation." Accessed January 8, 2017. www.arthritis.org/living-with-arthritis /arthritis-diet/foods-to-avoid-limit /food-ingredients-and-inflammation.php.

Berthet, Catherine. "Steps Toward a Better Anti-Inflammatory Lifestyle." *Palo Alto Medical Foundation*. August 2016. www.pamf.org/youngadults/health/diseases /Anti-Inflammatory-Pamphlet.pdf.

Bordoni, A., F. Danesi, D. Dardevet, D. Dupont, A. S. Fernandez, D. Gille, C. N. Dos Santos, et al. "Dairy Products and Inflammation: A Review of the Clinical Evidence." *Critical Reviews in Food Science and Nutrition* (August 2015). doi: 10.1080/10408398.2014.967385.

Calder, P. C., R. Albers, J-M. Antoine, S. Blum, R. Bourdet-Sicard, G. A. Ferns, G. Folkerts, et al. "Inflammatory Disease Processes and Interactions with Nutrition." *British Journal of Nutrition* 101 (2009): S1–S45. doi:10.1017 /S0007114509377867.

Cleveland Clinic. "Foods That Fight Inflammation—and Why You Need Them." June 12, 2012. my.clevelandclinic.org/health /transcripts/1395_foods-that-fight -inflammation-and-why-you-need-them.

Dietary Guidelines for Americans, 2015–2020. Accessed November 28, 2016. www.health.gov /dietaryguidelines/2015/guidelines/.

Franz, M. "Nutrition, Inflammation, and Disease." *Today's Dietitian*. February 2014. www.todaysdietitian.com /newarchives/020314p44.shtml.

Giugliano, D., A. Ceriello, and K. Esposito. "The Effects of Diet on Inflammation." *Journal of the American College of Cardiology* 48, no. 4 (August 2006): 677–85.

Harvard Health Letter. "Mindful Eating." February 2011. www.health.harvard.edu /staying-healthy/mindful-eating.

Lally, P., C. H. M. van Jaarsveld, H. W. Potts, and J. Wardle. "How Are Habits Formed: Modeling Habit Formation in the Real World." *European Journal of Social Psychology* 40 (July 2009): 998–1009. doi:10.1002/ejsp.674.

Mercola, J. "New Study: Daily Walk Can Add 7 Years to Your Life." Accessed November 29, 2016. fitness.mercola.com/sites/fitness/archive/2015/09/11/daily-walk-benefits.aspx#_edn1.

Palmer, Sharon, "Inflammation: Can't Stand the Heat? Then Get in the Kitchen." *Today's Dietitian*. February 2011. www.todaysdietitian.com/newarchives/020911p36.shtml.

Reblin, M., and B. N. Uchino. (2008). "Social and Emotional Support and Its Implication for Health." *Current Opinion in Psychiatry* 21(2) 201–205. doi: 10.1097/YCO.0b013e3282f3ad89.

Sass, Cynthia, "Six Fascinating Things a Food Journal Can Teach You about Your Eating Habits." Accessed November 29, 2016. news. http://www.health.com/nutrition/6-fascinating-things-a-food-journal-can-teach-you-about-your-eating-habits.

Schindler, T. H., J. Cardenas, J. O. Prior, A. D. Facta, M. C. Kreissl, X. L. Zhang, J. Sayre. "Relationship between Increasing Body Weight, Insulin Resistance, Inflammation, Adipocytokine Leptin, and Coronary Circulatory Function." *Journal of the American College of Cardiology* 47, no. 6 (March 2006): 1188–95.

van der Vaart, H., D. S. Postma, W. Timmens, and N. H. T. Ten Hacken. "Acute Effects of Cigarette Smoke on Inflammation and Oxidative Stress: A Review. *Thorax* 59, no. 8 (2004): 713–21. doi:10.1136/thx.2003.012468.

Weil, Andrew, "Anti-Inflammatory Diet Tips." youtube.com/watch?v=SYmb0DYRQKQ.

Weil, Andrew. *Eating Well for Optimal Health*. New York: Random House, 2011.

Wu, S., Shu, X., Chow, W. "Soy Food Intake and Circulating Levels of Inflammatory Markers in Chinese Women." *Journal of the Academy of Nutrition and Dietetics*. 112, no. 7 (July 2012), 996–1004. doi: 10.1016/j.jand.2012.04.001.

RECIPE INDEX

INDEX

ACKNOWLEDGMENTS

Lulu's Acknowledgments

For Tanya Smith, whose patience and support for my distraction while I was in the midst of moving around the world was unending. Also for Ace Noel, the teen who provides reality checks on every suggestion I think is helpful and wise—she does not always agree, and that makes my writing better. Everything I know about nutrition started with Dr. Marjorie Freedman, and any expertise I have in the practical truth of it was honed under the supervision of Terri Brownlee, MS, RDN. They both have my lifelong gratitude. My co-author Dorothy Calimeris was a blast to trade ideas with, and she made it fun to write this book. Finally, my path of learning about and ultimately loving food was supported at every step by my mother, Judy, who did not make as many healthful choices as I hope our readers will. Wish you could have seen this book published, Mama.

Dorothy's Acknowledgments

I'd like to thank my husband, Bob, my daughter, Claire, and all my family and friends who frequent my table. Additionally, I'd like to thank my students who continue to inspire me to find simple, effective ways to teach them how to cook and eat well. Last I'd like to thank my editor, Clara Song Lee, for putting up with me for the last three books. Her patience and grace are enviable. And a shout-out to the entire Callisto Media team.

ABOUT THE AUTHORS

LULU COOK is a registered dietitian nutrition-ist with expertise in sustainable food systems and holistic health. She promotes the power of a whole foods, plant-based diet to support a healthy environment and vibrant well-being for people at every stage of life. By working with individuals at farmers' markets, eating disor-der and substance abuse recovery programs, corporate wellness centers, and skilled nursing facilities, she has developed a broad under-standing of the challenges people face in making positive choices a foundation in their lives. Lulu is an enthusiastic and occasionally suc-cessful gardener, currently living and coaching in Brisbane, Australia. Reach her on Twitter @DhammaDish.

DOROTHY CALIMERIS is a food writer and blogger, and a frequent contributor to *Diablo* magazine. She is co-author of the bestselling cookbook *The Anti-Inflammatory Diet and Action Plans* and *The Good Life Mediterranean Diet Cookbook*, as well as a recipe developer and culinary instructor. Dorothy lives in Oakland, California, with her husband and daughter, and spends her days thinking about what she wants to eat next. Learn more at dorothyeats.com.

CPSIA information can be obtained
at www.ICGtesting.com
Printed in the USA
BVHW01s1934021117
499067BV00002B/2/P